COPING WITH
HIGH
BLOOD
PRESSURE

COPING WITH HIGH BLOOD PRESSURE

by Sandy Sorrentino, M.D., Ph.D.
and Carl Hausman

Foreword by Patricia Neal

*National Chairperson,
Patricia Neal Rehabilitation Center*

DEMBNER BOOKS • NEW YORK

Dembner Books
Published by Red Dembner Enterprises Corp., 80 Eighth Avenue, New York, N.Y. 10011
Distributed by W. W. Norton & Company, Inc., 500 Fifth Avenue, New York, N.Y. 10110

Illustrations in Chapter 1 are used with the kind permission of Craig Zuckerman.

Library of Congress Cataloging-in-Publication Data

Sorrentino, Sandy.
    Coping with high blood pressure.

    Includes index.
      1. Hypertension—Popular works.   I. Hausman, Carl,
1953–   .   II. Title.
RC685.H8S644   1986   616.1'32   86-6239
ISBN 0-934878-76-5
ISBN 0-942637-25-9 (pbk.)

Contents

Foreword

In 1965, a stroke changed my life. It meant a long and difficult period of recovery—a time that was trying for me and for my family and friends.

Unfortunately, strokes continue to change people's lives. Stroke is the nation's leading cause of disability and the third leading cause of death.

Controlling your blood pressure is a critical factor in heading off strokes, as well as in prevention of heart and kidney disease.

Coping with High Blood Pressure shows you how to get control of hypertension. This book offers readable explanations of the effects of high blood pressure and explores the ways you and your doctor can use medications and nondrug therapy to keep a lid on your blood pressure. It also includes comprehensive programs for physical fitness, diet, and stress reduction.

I strongly urge anyone with high blood pressure to do something about the problem now: Lowering your pressure is a key weapon in winning the battle against stroke. And that battle *is* being won. At the Patricia Neal Rehabilitation Center at the Fort Sanders Regional Medical Center in Knoxville, we are helping many stroke victims overcome their disabilities and get on with their lives.

It goes without saying, however, that preventing an illness is a far better alternative than recovering from one. So please take this opportunity to take control of your blood pressure and of your life.

Patricia Neal
Patricia Neal Rehabilitation Center
Fort Sanders Regional Medical Center
Knoxville, Tennessee

To Marie and Susan

Introduction

We know who you are. Because you have picked up this book in the first place, it is likely that you:

- were once diagnosed as having high blood pressure, but stopped taking your medication because it produced intolerable side effects. You are concerned about the effects of ignoring the problem.
- are taking your medicine despite the side effects, but you are unhappy with the treatment program and wonder if a better drug could be found, or the dosage reduced, or drug therapy eliminated altogether.
- do not know if you have high blood pressure or not—and no one else seems to, either. Perhaps you were once diagnosed as having high blood pressure (at a health fair, maybe) but found your blood pressure back to normal the next time it was checked. Or maybe one health care professional told you your reading was high but another maintained that the reading was normal—even though it was the *same* reading. What's the story here? It is a question that has been bothering you for some time now.
- have already suffered some damage from high blood pressure, such as a stroke or heart attack, and your doctor has told you to get that pressure down *now*.

Pretty close, aren't we? Well, there's no magic in this diagnosis because *there are millions of people in the same situation*. High blood pressure is one of the most confused and confusing areas of medicine—to both the layman and to the physician. One reason is that research

11

findings and new medications change the picture frequently. Secondly, science has yet to unlock all the mysteries of the body's function; there is no universal agreement among physicians as to the precise causes of high blood pressure or even as to how high a reading translates to "high" blood pressure.

From your standpoint, the treatment factor is another important variable. Drugs for treatment of hypertension have traditionally been known for their wide variety of side effects, most of them unpleasant, and some dangerous. However, new drugs and new strategies for administering those drugs have considerably reduced the likelihood of unbearable side effects. It is quite possible, too, that you recieved unskilled or indifferent care in the prescription of drugs for high blood pressure. To be candid, far too many physicians have adopted a mechanical approach to treatment and have prescribed drugs that may not precisely fit the problem *or the patient*.

So which is your scenario? Did you drop out of drug therapy because it was difficult to take a pill that made you feel miserable—especially since you had felt perfectly fine despite high blood pressure? We will help you try again, because new treatment approaches combined with your knowledge can overcome the problem.

Did you ignore one report of high blood pressure because the next reading was lower, or because another doctor said your pressure was not high enough to treat? This book will spell out the newly discovered dangers of blood pressure that bounces up and down, and will explain why even a slight degree of high blood pressure is worthy of prompt attention.

Are you curious about the potentials of drug-free therapy? It may or may not be a possibility in your case, but you and your doctor may decide that weight loss, exercise, and stress reduction are worth a try.

In any event, high blood pressure *must* be treated. It is an insidious, vicious killer, and we are not saying this just to sell books.

It is one of the most serious health problems in the United States.

It is one of the least understood.

And it is one of the most responsive to treatment.

* * *

The risks of high blood pressure and the relevant mechanics of your body will be explained in Chapter 1. The ways in which treatments fail—a major problem for physicians and patients—will be outlined in Chapter 2.

Chapter 3 gives a short course in drugs for treatment of high blood pressure; it talks about their effects, side effects, and what you can do to make your treatment plan workable *for you.*

Not all people, however, need drug treatments. Some of us can use drug-free strategies to control high blood pressure. The methods of lowering blood pressure through diet, exercise, and stress reduction can also help those who do need drugs from eventually requiring more potent (and side-effect-ridden) medications. The drug-free lowering of blood pressure will be addressed in Chapters 4, 5, 6, and 7.

Chapter 8 will address some special problems, such as high blood pressure in children, the elderly, blacks, or those suffering from compounding conditions or illnesses. Because new and exciting treatments are being discovered with great regularity, Chapter 9 will discuss advances on the horizon and give you a groundwork from which to evaluate what you hear and read in the press.

The final chapter deals with lifelong blood pressure control, and helps you work with your doctor to set your personal treatment goals.

Coping with High Blood Pressure will not qualify you to hang out your own shingle, but it certainly will help make you an informed patient. And when it comes to controlling high blood pressure, that is very, very important.

Why? Because it is your responsibility to take control of this illness. Your doctor cannot make sure you take your pills or control your diet. In point of fact, your doctor or doctors may provide poor, uncoordinated, or inconsistent care. In that situation, it is up to you to ask about changing a treatment program that does not seem to work.

High blood pressure is dangerous, and it is up to you to take that responsibility *now.* So—please—turn the page and let's get started.

[1]
Blood Pressure—
What It Is and
Why It Matters

The following are true cases. The names are fictitious.

- Frank's blood pressure problem was solved permanently on New Year's Day. The fifty-one-year-old businessman will no longer have to contend with the fact that his blood pressure medicine made him urinate frequently (which is why he stopped taking it). A massive heart attack wiped out a major portion of his heart muscle, meaning that the heart will never again have the strength to produce a high blood pressure. "There's not much we can do for Frank," the physician informed the family. "What we can do is to start studying his children for high blood pressure. It's not too late for them—but it's too bad the point has to be made this way."
- Madeline's blood pressure had been high for more than thirty years. Because she had followed her corporate-executive husband from city to city, Madeline had seen a number of doctors but never received consistent monitoring. Each doctor noted that the blood pressure was relatively high, and Madeline always promised to lose weight, cut back on salt, and check in again in a few months. She never did. On a rainy June day, the sixty-eight-year-old was admitted to the hospital because she complained of persistent weakness. The physician noted that her blood pressure was quite high and suspected kidney damage, one typical result of untreated blood pressure. Test results painted a grim picture: Madeline's kidney function was 50 percent destroyed. "This means," he told the frightened woman, "that your body can't filter out its own poisons, and you may have to go on dialysis."
- Don was thirty-five, healthy-looking and feeling fine. During an insurance physical, a doctor noted that Don's blood pressure was alarmingly high. The doctor prescribed a powerful drug that, among other effects, once interfered with Don's ability to have an erection. The pills went into the drawer and Don went on with his

17

life, which included generous doses of drinking, heavy eating, and gambling. He continued to feel perfectly well.

His first symptom was sudden death: a massive stroke during sex with a prostitute.

If you think the above cases are scare tactics, you are right. Who would not be scared of a disease that produces no symptoms but can destroy the heart, the arteries, the brain, the kidneys, and the eyes? By the time the damage is detected, it is generally permanent.

Understanding the Silent Killer

High blood pressure is known as the silent killer, with good reason. It can take years to develop, years to do the damage, it is generally painless, and by the time the first symptoms appear, the only alternative often is to wheel in the heart-lung machines, the dialysis units, or call the brain surgeon.

Physicians know that most high blood pressure can be controlled, long before the stages where heroic measures must be taken to preserve the fading function of the heart, kidneys, or other organs. That is why doctors frequently feel the urge to grab a high-blood-pressure patient by the lapels and read the riot act.

But patients are often blind (as mentioned, a literal consequence of high blood pressure) to the facts. One of the most important reasons people ignore the problem is that the whole concept of blood pressure is somewhat abstract. A "bad heart" commands instant attention, but "high blood pressure" does not seem to fire up the same alarm bells. And how high is high, anyway? When does one become alarmed?

Another factor that blunts reaction to high blood pressure is that people really do have a difficult time believing a disease that produces no symptoms can kill them.

We will deal with both of those concepts in this chapter. A clear understanding of what blood pressure is will give you a better picture of how normal blood pressure goes out of control. This knowledge will be more immediately useful when we discuss how various treatments lower blood pressure.

And the discussion of what high blood pressure does to your organs and how it does this dirty work will, we hope, certainly motivate you to act.

What Is Blood Pressure?

First, let's demystify the concept of blood pressure. Blood pressure, BP for short, is the pressure of the blood in the body's arterial system. The arterial system carries oxygen-rich blood away from the heart and into the tissues. The arteries branch off into smaller vessels called arterioles, which in turn branch off into capillaries, tiny vessels only one blood-cell wide.

After the blood has delivered oxygen and nutrients to the cells, it enters the veins, which transport the blood back to the heart and lungs.

The pressure in the arteries and arterioles (not the veins) is what is important in high blood pressure. To better picture what happens in the artery, let's examine how blood pressures are taken and what the numbers indicate.

A physician or health professional uses a device called a sphygmomanometer to measure BP. This instrument is much easier to use than to pronounce.

First, the cuff is wrapped around the patient's arm and tightened by means of a pump that inflates the cuff and cuts off most of the circulation in the arm. A valve then is released, allowing air to seep out and the cuff to loosen.

The doctor places a stethoscope over the artery located in the crook of the elbow. When the cuff becomes loose enough for the blood to spurt through the artery, the doctor hears the turbulence through the stethoscope and notes the reading on the sphygmomanometer's dial. (The rushing of the blood sounds like *pshht . . . pshht . . . pshht . . .* and is known as the Korotkoff sound.)

That reading indicates the *systolic* pressure. The systolic pressure means the pressure of the blood in the arteries *as the heart beats* (that is, when it contracts).

Now, the doctor continues releasing pressure from the cuff until the turbulent sounds disappear. When the sounds disappear, he notes the reading on the dial. That reading is the *diastolic* pressure. The diastolic pressure indicates the pressure in the arteries *when the heart is at rest* (not contracted).

The BP is expressed in terms of the systolic over the diastolic pressure. (The first word relates to the *systole*, which means the part of the heart's cycle when it pumps; *diastole* is the phase where it rests and fills with blood.) Actual numbers indicate the reading in terms of millimeters (mm) of mercury (Hg), a measurement that indicates how high the pressure would raise a specifically designed column of mercury.

So, the reading might be registered as:

$$\frac{120 \text{ mm Hg (systolic)}}{80 \text{ mm Hg (diastolic)}}$$

And would be expressed in speech as "one-twenty over eighty," or "120/80" in writing. 120/80 is a normal reading; BP is consisdered normal up to about 140/90. Above that, the reading is considered to indicate high blood pressure, or *hypertension*, a word that means exactly the same thing and which we will use from now on to indicate high blood pressure. A person with high blood pressure is said by physicians to be *hypertensive*.

What Is High Blood Pressure?

The degree of hypertension, along with other factors, will determine what the physician does about the condition. In some cases, changes in diet or physical condition will suffice. (Exactly how and why diet and conditioning affect blood pressure will be explained later in this book.) For more severe hypertension, drug treatments will be necessary. The potency of the drug will depend on the degree of hypertension and, to an extent, the underlying cause.

Here are how the varying degrees are generally categorized. As mentioned earlier, not all physicians will agree on what levels require which types of treatment, but the classifications are pretty much universally agreed to.

Borderline	140/90	The majority of hypertensives fall into this
(also referred	to 160/104	category. Often, borderline hypertensives can
to as "mild")		be treated effectively with diet, salt reduction,
		and weight control.

Moderate	160/104 to 190/115	Danger of damage to organs (such as damage to arteries, heart, and kidneys, explained more fully later in this chapter) is increased, but the type of treatment may vary with the individual. For instance, the physician might take into account a recent weight gain by a young man just married. In this case, there is a chance that the dietary problem will level itself out. But in another case, a heavy drinker who has shown little evidence of self-care in the past is not a good candidate for dietary restriction, and would more likely benefit from drug therapy.
Severe	190/115 and above, no symptoms	Severe hypertension warrants immediate examination for organ damage and prescription of a potent antihypertensive medication.
Crisis	190/115 and above, with symptoms	A hypertensive crisis is severe hypertension with accompanying symptoms, such as dizziness, headache, and seizures. Immediate emergency intervention is essential.

Again, the question arises: How high is high? Since the majority of hypertension falls into the borderline area, the question has great validity, and leads into the broader questions of the effects and causes of hypertension.

The Dangers of Hypertension

The examples presented at the opening of this chapter give an idea of the severity of the problem on an individual basis. But let's take a look at some of the facts as they relate to the statistical risks that you, the hypertensive, are encountering right now as you read this page.

First of all, consider the fact that you have a lot of company. About one in five Americans has some degree of hypertension. Sadly, that hypertension contributes directly to an estimated million deaths a year through heart attack, stroke, or kidney disease.

Now, let's return to the "how high is high" question as it relates to borderline hypertension, a problem that affects maybe twenty million

Americans. Insurance actuarial data says that even this mild, borderline hypertension contributes significantly to morbidity and mortality (physicians' words for sickness and death). One major insurance company, for example, reports that the life expectancy of a thirty-five-year-old man can.be reduced by about sixteen years if his blood pressure is 150/100 compared to 120/80.

If that frightens you—well, hold on because it gets worse. A hypertensive's chance of getting a stroke is four times higher than a normotensive (a person with normal BP). One famous study, conducted in Framingham, Massachusetts, showed that heart attacks are three to four times more likely to strike a hypertensive than a normotensive.

We can trot out more statistics but you certainly have got the point. Even a mild elevation in blood pressure is dangerous, and the risks increase drastically with an increase in the degree of hypertension or in the length of time hypertension has had to pound away at your arteries and organs.

In short, we can say something about hypertension that is very rare in the medical and scientific fields: It has been proven *almost* conclusively that hypertension is deadly.

The qualification in the above sentence is part of the language of science, and reflects something you should be aware of when dealing with any medical issue. In the strictly structured world of scientific research, it is one thing to show a statistical linkage between two factors—say, high blood pressure and stroke—and quite another to say that high blood pressure *caused* the stroke.

In science, there are very few cases where an ironclad chain of events can be established to prove, for example, that smoking causes cancer, or that exercise increases life span, or even that high blood pressure contributes to disease. What we rely on are *epidemiologic* data, which are records of what happened to whom. We have to make the best suppositions we can based on the evidence.

We bring up this rather cumbersome point because you may encounter occasional studies that seem to debunk the linkage between high blood pressure and a malady like coronary artery disease. (An actual study did make this assertion.) When dealing with information of this type, remember that hypertension is a slow-acting disease and the effects may not surface until thirty years after the end of the study, an occurrence that could certainly distort the results.

Too, bear in mind that, for reasons of medical ethics, physicians often will not set up what is known as a control group, a group of subjects that would be monitored but *not* treated, in order to observe the progress of a disease if there is no medical intervention. However, the lack of a strictly enforced control group may affect results significantly.

Thirdly, consider the fact that hypertension is a disease colored by virtually everything that people do in their lifetime. It is extraordinarily difficult to sort out the effects of diet, physical condition, mental state—and the interaction of all three—when compiling data.

The point is that although some minor studies might indicate otherwise, the evidence is overwhelming that hypertension, even relatively mild hypertension, is dangerous.

To make matters worse, hypertension is easy to ignore. Some studies show that half of hypertensives do not know they have the disease, and of the ones who do, only half bother to get treatment.

As we have stated (but cannot state too often), hypertension does its damage without symptoms. To understand what happens, it is worthwhile to take a quick look at how hypertension comes about and what happens once it does.

The Causes of Hypertension

The majority of hypertension falls into the category of *essential* hypertension, also called *primary* or *idiopathic* hypertension. The three terms mean basically the same thing: that the hypertension is not directly caused by another identifiable cause or is without an immediately identifiable cause. To translate the medical jargon, primary and essential and idiopathic, as related to hypertension, mean we just don't know what causes it.

Sometimes a direct cause is found, and those relatively rare cases are classified as *secondary hypertension*.

Essential Hypertension

There are many theories about the cause of essential hypertension. The most basic suppositions involve the incredibly complex system the body uses to balance its functions. Hypertension occurs when these systems somehow go out of whack. Essential hypertension is a failure of the self-regulatory mechanism and is probably hereditary.

It was once thought that higher blood pressure was a normal, in fact a desirable, consequence of aging. When arteries hardened, it was reasoned, more pressure was needed to force the blood through them. However, subsequent research showed that hardening of the arteries was more a phenomenon *caused* by hypertension—but more about that later.

Assuming that hypertension is a system out of kilter, where does the fault lie? A link-by-link tour through the chain of interacting systems can begin in the *baroreceptors*, sensors in the walls of arteries that feel a pressure that is too high and send a signal through the nervous system to the heart, instructing it to slow down, and also signal the muscular walls of the arterioles to relax.

That is one way in which the body balances its blood pressure. Remember, though, that there are times when the body wants its blood pressure to be high: dangerous situations where it is vital to fight or flee, for example, when the body needs increased circulation. You are probably familiar with *adrenaline*, the substance that triggers rapid heart beat and, in effect, prepares the body for fight or flight. Adrenaline is secreted by the adrenal glands, which are located above the kidneys. Adrenaline, also known as *epinephrine*, increases heart rate and blood pressure and constricts the arterioles. One theory holds that this is an ancient instinctive reaction to control bleeding in a battle.

The baroreceptors and the nervous system are one factor in the delicate blood-pressure balance. Adrenaline—which is a substance known as a hormone—is another. A third factor is *renin*. Renin is an enzyme secreted by the kidneys. Its purpose is to keep blood pressure from dropping too low.

Renin does this by teaming up with another substance produced in the liver and forming a substance called *angiotensin I*. Angiotensin I is turned into a substance called *angiotensin II* by a substance called, appropriately, an *angiotensin-converting enzyme*, or *ACE*. Angiotensin II is the real villain here, as it is a powerful constrictor of the arterioles.

(OK, you are confused. Unfortunately, there is no easy way to explain this. Hang on for a couple more paragraphs—at least remember the names of the substances—and you will be several steps closer to understanding essential hypertension and how it eventually is treated.) When angiotensin II constricts the arterioles, it does so by forcing extra calcium into the arterioles. Calcium causes the constriction, a point that will become important when we consider the various medicinal ways of reducing hypertension.

Angiotensin II also signals the adrenal gland to produce a hormone called aldosterone, which causes the kidney to retain sodium. Sodium, in turn, causes the body to retain water. An increase in water translates to an increase in the amount of blood, hence higher pressure.

When the body's system of checks and balances is in working order, the production of blood-pressure-increasing substances is stopped when blood pressure reaches what the body thinks is an adequate level, appropriate for the current situation. Adrenaline production is stopped when the fight-or-flight situation is over. The kidney stops pumping out renin when it senses that an adequate blood flow to the kidney has been restored.

But for some of us, the signals go awry and those body systems do not shut down. The result is essential hypertension. As we will see in following chapters, diet, physical condition, drugs, and a combination of these elements can be used to throw the off-switch on an out-of-control system.

Secondary Hypertension

Another compelling reason to see a physician if you suspect high blood pressure (perhaps because of a family history of the disease) is to rule out directly related medical causes. It is possible—but not likely, as we have already noted—that your hypertension is secondary to another condition. ("Secondary to" is medical terminology for "caused by.")

Some possible causes of secondary hypertension are:

- *Primary hyperaldosteronism.* A tumor on the adrenal gland causes a runaway increase in the level of aldosterone. Treatment involves surgical removal of the tumor.
- *Pheochromocytoma.* This is also a tumor in the adrenal gland, but a pheochromocytoma causes runaway formation of adrenaline and another hormone called noradrenaline. It increases the force of the

heart's pumping action and also causes blood vessel constriction. Treatment involves surgical removal of the tumor.

- *Renal artery disease.* When the artery feeding the kidney is blocked, the kidney pumps out renin (as discussed above). This activates the chain of events that raises BP. Surgical removal of the blockage can often alleviate the problem.
- *Narrowing of the aorta.* The aorta, the main artery carrying blood from the heart to the rest of the body, sometimes is narrow at birth. This so-called *coarctation* requires more pressure in order for the blood to pass. As a result, the blood pressure throughout the body is increased. The coarctation can usually be repaired surgically.
- *Other causes.* Less common causes of secondary hypertension include Cushing's disease (a disease causing overproduction of certain hormones), brain tumors, anemia, certain kidney diseases and inflammations, and use of birth control pills.

The diagnosis of secondary hypertension involves use of tests such as an intravenous pyelogram (for evaluation of kidney and kidney artery function) and chest X-rays (looking for symptoms of coarctation of the aorta). These tests are ordered only if the physical examination indicates initial evidence of secondary causes.

As you have probably figured out, diagnosing essential hypertension is largely a matter of ruling out other possible causes. And, in about nine out of ten cases, those causes *will* be ruled out and the business of controlling essential hypertension will begin.

The Effects of Hypertension

Why bother to control hypertension? We have discussed some of the statistics, and the numbers make a compelling argument. But even more convincing is a close examination of the damage done to organs.

Here is a quick tour of the vital organs—and a graphic description of what hypertension does to them.

The Arteries

For reasons that are not completely clear, hypertension hastens hardening of the arteries, a process known as *arteriosclerosis* or

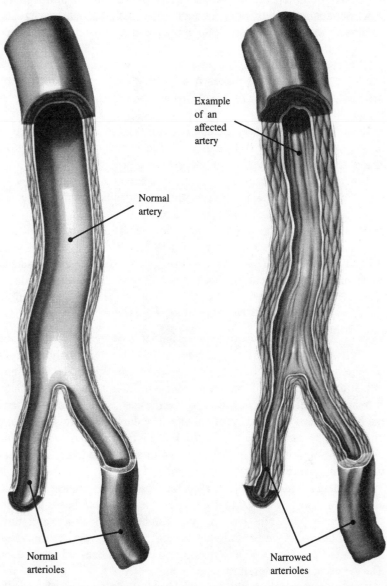

Example
of an
affected
artery

Normal
artery

Normal
arterioles

Narrowed
arterioles

Figure 1. Normal Blood Pressure   **Figure 2.** High Blood Pressure

atherosclerosis. The terms are basically synonymous, although arteriosclerosis is the broader category and includes atherosclerosis. Atherosclerosis refers to a buildup of plaque on the inside lining, called the *intima,* of the artery.

One theory holds that the increased pressure of the blood flow damages the intima and makes it more susceptible to narrowing by deposits of plaque and cholesterol. (More about cholesterol in Chapter 5.)

Regardless of the cause, the end result is a narrowing of the bore of the artery (Figures 1 and 2), with a subsequent reduction of blood flow and a resulting aggravation of the pressure problem.

The location where atherosclerotic disease appears determines its precise impact. In coronary arteries, the result can be angina (explained in a moment) or a heart attack. If atherosclerotic narrowing of the arteries occurs in the brain, stroke can result. In kidneys, atherosclerosis can result in a reduction of the organs' filtering capabilities. As will be shown, the eyes are also susceptible. Hypertension also has some effect on the hearing mechanism.

Hypertension and the Heart

Hypertension forces the heart to pump harder in order to force the blood through narrowed arteries. As a result, the heart actually enlarges (Figure 3). It increases in thickness because of the additional stress and also stretches because of the larger volume of fluid it must accomodate.

When the heart stretches too far, the muscle tissue is damaged and the heart no longer pumps as efficiently. The damage is irreversible and unfortunately can easily be overlooked in a routine physical if no electrocardiogram is taken. Once symptoms are noticed, a great deal of damage may already have been done.

Hypertension is especially related to a type of heart disease known as *congestive heart failure.* In this case, the enlarged heart loses its capability to push blood out of its chambers, and as a result fluid pressure builds up on the left side of the heart. The veins can not take this kind of pressure, and as a result fluid is forced back into the lungs. The heart may never return to normal.

Angina (pronounced either AN-gin-uh or an-JIGH-nuh) literally means "heart pain." It is caused by a lack of blood flow to the heart,

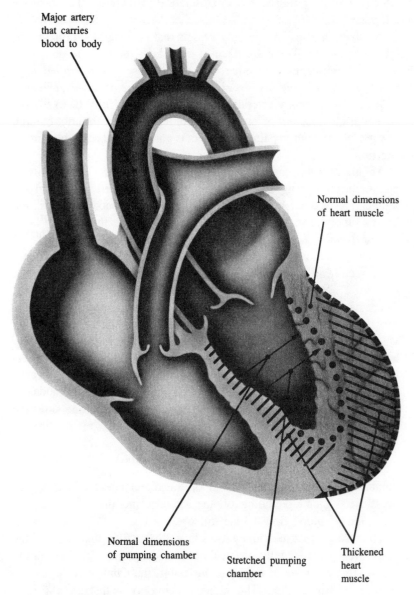

Major artery
that carries
blood to body

Normal dimensions
of heart muscle

Normal dimensions
of pumping chamber

Stretched pumping
chamber

Thickened
heart
muscle

Figure 3. Some Possible (but Preventable) Effects on the Heart

which in turn is caused by atherosclerotic disease of the coronary arteries.

Coronary arteries are the only vessels that provide blood directly to the heart muscle. There are three of them and, for some reason, they are highly susceptible to atherosclerotic disease. *Uncontrolled high blood pressure is the biggest risk factor in coronary artery disease.*

When the coronary arteries become partially or fully blocked, the heart muscle does not receive enough blood and therefore not enough oxygen. It cries out in pain. This effect is particularly noticeable during exertion.

Angina is often described as a squeezing, crushing discomfort or pain in the chest. Angina itself can be crippling in severe cases, and it is a precursor of other heart disease. If the blockage becomes acute, the heart's supply of oxygen will be cut off. The result is the death of heart muscle tissue—a heart attack.

An important related point: Recent research indicates that about one-third of all heart attacks are so-called silent heart attacks, meaning that they were not recognized as heart attacks at the time they occurred. Silent heart attacks are very often found in hypertensive individuals. Most silent heart attacks are discovered during electrocardiograms, where the tracings will indicate past damage. That is one reason why having an EKG (electrocardiogram—the reason it is abbreviated E*K*G is because the term was taken from the German spelling) is so important. If nothing else, it establishes a baseline from which your physician can determine if any silent damage has been done since the time of the last exam.

Hypertension and the Kidneys

Nephrosclerosis is a combination of the direct effect of the highly pressurized blood pounding on the kidneys and the atherosclerotic reduction of blood flow to the kidneys.

The result is that the kidney loses its ability to filter toxins out of the body. Most victims of this problem have no symptoms until they start to retain large amounts of fluid. At this point, the damage is difficult to reverse or irreversible. The kidneys can only withstand a certain amount of stress before they wear out. When they wear out, they will not regenerate and dialysis may be the only answer. And when kidneys are damaged, they often cause blood pressure to increase further, a vicious cycle.

Kidney disease is a particularly unpleasant fate, and is a tragic price to pay for untreated hypertension.

Hypertension and the Brain

One effect of hypertension is known as *acute hypertensive encephalopathy*, a swelling of the brain and a short-circuiting of the nervous pathways. The patient requires immediate emergency treatment with powerful pharmacological agents. This condition typically affects someone with long-term blood pressure problems who has been negligent in self-care.

Here is a typical case history: One night, after an evening out with the boys (drinking raises blood pressure) and a clambake (a lot of salty food), several cups of coffee and a pack of cigarettes, the BP goes out of sight and the brain just cannot handle the rapid rise. If treated in time, the brain can be returned to normal. If not, brain injury or death may result.

Another type of brain injury linked to hypertension is an *intracranial hemorrhage*, one type of stroke. This is usually, though not always, a disease of the older adult who has had longstanding hypertension. Typically, the victim is on his or her feet, and suddenly is gripped by a violent headache, falls down, and is comatose within seconds. What has happened is that a damaged vessel has ruptured and leaked into the brain (Figure 4).

A more common type of stroke (called a thrombotic stroke) occurs when a damaged vessel becomes so narrowed that blood cannot flow to a section of the brain (Figure 5), and artery blockage results.

A third type of stroke linked to high blood pressure occurs when an area of atherosclerotic artery roughens, allowing blood to clot on it. When the blood clot breaks loose, it lodges in a smaller artery. This is known as an *embolus*, and when it occurs in the brain, it can result in death of a portion of this organ (called an embolic stroke).

Incidentally, new evidence points out that the brain has its own type of angina: a condition known as a *transient ischemic attack*, or TIA.

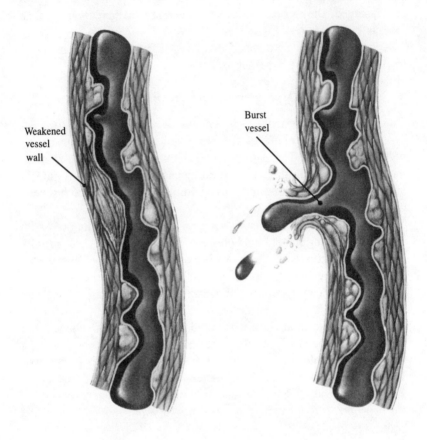

Figure 4. Brain Hemorrhage, One Type of Stroke

(*Ischemic* means lacking oxygen.) A TIA patient appears to have had a stroke (for example, cannot speak normally) but reverts to normal in twenty-four hours. That time frame is the arbitrary definition of a TIA. A TIA is thought to result from small emboli (plural of embolus) thrown into the brain. While a TIA by definition does not cause permanent damage, it seems to be a precursor of future problems and apparently has a relationship to hypertension.

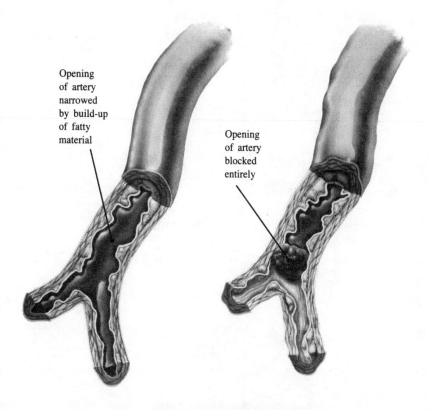

Opening
of artery
narrowed
by build-up
of fatty
material

Opening
of artery
blocked
entirely

Figure 5. Artery Blockage

Hypertension and the Eye

Here, the damage is atherosclerotic. An ophthalmologist looking into a healthy eye sees a pattern of blood vessels such as that pictured in Figure 6. Uncontrolled high blood pressure, though, produces a twisting and narrowing effect, cutting off some of the eye's blood supply (Figure 7).

Ischemia in the eye damages the retina, resulting in a variety of vision problems, including so-called tunnel vision.

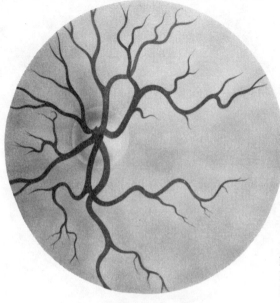

Figure 6. Normal
Blood Vessels
in the Eye

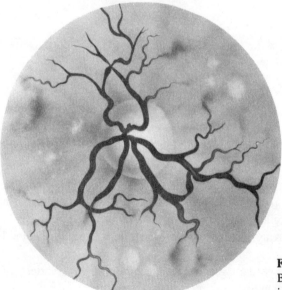

Figure 7. Damaged
Blood Vessels
in the Eye

The Long-term Killer

In sum, hypertension is more than a silent killer; it is a sneaky killer, creating no symptoms until the damage is done. It is a long-term killer, doing its damage over years, over decades.

Treating high blood pressure is indeed, as the American Heart Association says, a death-defying act. There is probably no one single action you can take, short of quitting cigarettes, that will have such a positive effect on your health.

Unfortunately, treatment is not always successful. The next chapter discusses how high blood pressure is diagnosed and treated—and why those treatments are not always as effective as they could be.

First, let's discuss some of the more frequently asked questions relating to the topics covered in this chapter.

Q: I have heard that the diastolic reading is the most important number—that the systolic varies with emotion and activity, but the diastolic really is what I should be concerned about. True?

A: Not really. Many studies, including the Framingham study, show that the upper reading is just as significant as the lower one.

Q: You mentioned that obesity is a factor in high blood pressure. Why is it?

A: The question will be examined more thoroughly in Chapter 5, but the essential fact is that the obese person's greater fluid volume causes an increase in blood pressure. Also, Chapter 5 will discuss how obesity is linked to the presence of cholesterol and other fatty substances in the blood.

Q: I have heard high blood pressure described as malignant hypertension? What kind is that?

A: Malignant hypertension is a special form of hypertension where blood pressure levels go wildly out of control. It is relatively rare. Physicians, as a rule, like to avoid this term because it implies that nonmalignant hypertension—benign hypertension—is harmless. Benign hypertension, while technically a correct term, is highly misleading to the layman.

[2]
Why Treatment
Fails

In the old days—which really were not so long ago—the physician treating a hypertensive patient might simply reach routinely into his black bag and pick out a drug—the drug he used as a first choice for all hypertensives. If the drug did not work, he would move on to the next more potent medicine—again, the same pills he used for all patients who did not respond to the first drug.

To be fair, this method was not always a result of laziness, nor did all doctors take such a mechanical approach to the prescription of antihypertensive medication. First of all, it was and is extremely difficult to keep up with new drugs and treatment approaches. The amount of new information that crosses a physician's desk is staggering, and those doctors without the time or inclination to bone up on the latest antihypertensive medications would stick to their old stand-bys.

And old stand-bys do have a strong appeal to the physician. After all, he or she has worked with the drug, prescribed it to many patients, knows the side effects intimately, and is confident that the particular pill is not dangerous. A new drug requires effort and risk.

In the last five years, we have made tremendous inroads into the pharmacological treatment of high blood pressure. New drugs virtually fit the particular symptoms like a key into a lock. But we physicians do have to break some old habits, and old habits die hard.

The Stepped Care Approach

One such habit is our tendency to be a slave to a mechanical application of what is called *stepped care*, a program of increasingly potent treatment. Basically, stepped care is a structured method of trial and error, starting in some cases with nondrug therapy and continuing with small doses of less-potent drugs. Potency and dosage are increased until the condition being treated is controlled. Stepped care is used in treatment of a variety of conditions, hypertension being one of them.

Stepped care has not always worked well, and the blame must be shared by the system itself, the doctors who use it, and the patients who all too often do not comply with their treatments.

The Problem with Stepped Care

In theory, stepped care looks like a highly efficient method of treatment—and it is, unless the stepped program is adhered to at the expense of dismissing the individual needs of the client.

For example, the traditional stepwise approach to drug therapy in hypertension begins with a diuretic, a drug that flushes fluid out of the system. If a diuretic does not bring down the blood pressure, other drugs will be added. (Not substituted, generally, but added.) Farther down the line, for example, a drug would be used to open up the arteries; such a drug is called a vasodilator.

Today, that approach might be altered. Physicians now understand much more about the physiology of hypertension. All hypertension is not the same.

Let's look at Mary, age fifty-one. She is overweight, has a puffy face and swollen ankles. Mary loves to eat, particularly salty foods. Mary's hypertension should respond very well to diuretics along with dietary restriction, as she is probably retaining a gallon of excess fluid in her system.

Grant, age forty-five, is another story. He is a hard-driving, type-A personality. Diuretics may not be the answer for him. His problem is not so much fluid retention but vascular constriction. Other drugs that act directly to relax the constriction of the arterioles seem to be a better choice. Grant's doctor could—and probably would, today—skip over the initial step of prescribing diuretics and find the precise drug for the situation, the key for the lock.

So while physicians really do not have a complete understanding of the causes of essential hypertension, their growing knowledge about the illness itself enables better treatment. Basically, many hypertension cases are starting to fall into the categories of

a) volume—meaning excess fluid, like Mary.

b) vascular—meaning a clamping of the arterioles, like Grant.

Vascular problems may also relate to overproduction of renin, and/or too-rapid or too-forceful a heartbeat.

The two types of hypertension are not mutually exclusive, nor are they definitive. But they do provide a starting point from which to examine the issue, and as we will see in the material on antihypertensive medications, our increasing knowledge of the physiology of high blood pressure is allowing us to enter the hypertension cycle at various points. Lock-and-key drugs let the physician shut down the out-of-control regulatory system with the appropriate switch.

The Problem with Doctors

It is probably a fair statement to say that younger physicians in general have a better understanding of the physiology of hypertension than do older doctors. Once a doctor is out of training and into practice, he or she often gets further removed from new developments and research.

Doctors frequently do not have the time or take the time to keep up with research and new treatment programs. Where a younger physician has been trained in aggressive use of newer antihypertensive drugs, an older doctor must make an effort to master their use.

(Incidentally, this is not an indictment of age versus youth. Today's younger doctors will shortly be older doctors, farther removed from recent developments, etc. Nor is this true in every case; a great many older doctors assiduously keep up with research and new drugs.)

Typically, the doctor with little interest in and knowledge of hypertension control will try three or four mechanical steps, and if they do not work, he or she will ship the patient off to an expert.

Here is where the issue gets a bit clouded, because there are no "experts," per se, in the sense of a medical specialty. While you can flip the yellow pages and find physicians listed under such headings as nephrology (kidney), ophthalmology (eye), or gastroenterology (digestive tract), there is no specialty for hypertension. Indeed, there are no hospital training programs devoted specifically to hypertension.

The expert usually is a specialist in another field who has developed, purely on his or her own initiative, a strong interest in hypertension control. The specialist may be an internist, that is, a specialist who in a sense is a generalist; or a kidney specialist, who approaches the hypertension problem from the standpoint of renal function; or the specialist may even come from far-afield specialties such as endocrinology (hormone study).

Most doctors are aware of the physicians in their area who have developed an informal specialty in control of hypertension, and that is who you may eventually see if your family physician feels you would be better served by referral to the informal specialist.

Another point concerning you and your doctor: We will mention from time to time that if your program is not working out, you might seek a second opinion. Many times, patients do not do this for fear of offending their physician. In the case of hypertension, though, you may find your doctor is actually relieved that you will get another opinion.

Why? First of all, the field is advancing so rapidly that your doctor would welcome the contribution of additional knowledge. Secondly, to be perfectly candid, your doctor just might want you out of his or her hair. Hypertension is not a rewarding disease to treat, either from a professional or financial standpoint. Patients with a strep throat love their doctors. The patients come in feeling terrible, get some pills, and feel better in a day or so. Patients with high blood pressure come in feeling fine and frequently get pills that make them feel terrible. This is certainly not the kind of case many doctors enjoy managing, nor do they find it cost-effective in terms of their income. Time is money, and dealing with hypertension takes a lot of the doctor's time.

The Problem with Patients

From the physician's standpoint, the biggest problem in hypertension control lies with patient compliance—in other words, getting the patient to stay on a diet, exercise, and take the proper medications.

Many doctors view hypertension as a bubbling cauldron, a sinister brew of dietary, hereditary, and lifestyle factors. So not only does the doctor have to be a physician, he has to be a dietician and a psychologist as well.

And trying to get that witches' brew back down to a simmer is no easy job. The patient's life will probably be fundamentally changed in some way, whether from alterations in diet, lifestyle, or the addition of powerful medications. For example, it is not easy for patients to accept the fact that they:

- can never abuse salt again.
- should stop smoking.
- must revamp their diet to eliminate high-cholesterol, high-fat, and salty foods.
- should start an exercise program, if capable.
- should try to control stress.
- should lose weight.
- should control the use of alcohol and caffeine.

And this does not even bring into account the drugs that may or may not be necessary!

So, we have seen how the blood pressure situation is confused and confusing from a variety of standpoints, and how the ball is dropped on occasion by both physicians and patients. Maybe you have been the victim of a few fumbles yourself.

Let's see how hypertension treatment is supposed to work. Then we will look at how it sometimes goes wrong. After sorting out the successes and failures, you will have a better idea of what might be right for you.

Stepped Care When It Works

The key to effective management of hypertension is knowledge—and since it is ultimately up to you to keep the fire under that cauldron low, let's walk some hypothetical patients through the stepped care system. Remember two things during the trip:

1. Stepped care is not in and of itself bad medicine. It is the rigid adherence to inappropriate steps in the system that causes problems. Good treatment of hypertension will still be on the stepped approach, but the steps will be lock-and-key precise.
2. While the stepped care approach involves trial and error, the biggest error is usually made by the patient who does not stay on the treatment plan. The best program in the world does no good if you do not follow it.

What follows is stepped care when it works. It will illustrate the various stages and give a basic introduction to the broad categories of drug treatment. After this example, we will talk about how it can go wrong.

Step Zero

Patient A's blood pressure is high. Dr. Hypothetical, who is knowledgeable about these things, takes several readings. Because some patients develop high blood pressure just from the tension of being in the doctor's office, Dr. Hypothetical asks the patient to wait for a while before the second reading is taken.

Dr. Hypothetical also takes readings with the patient standing and sitting; readings are also taken in both arms. Several readings are useful because much hypertension is *labile*, meaning it bounces around quite a bit. (Labile hypertension will be addressed in greater detail in Chapter 8, which deals with special problems.)

A physical, which includes tests of kidney function and an examination of the eyes and heart, turns up no end-organ damage, so Dr. Hypothetical reads Patient A the riot act and sends him home to stew about it for a while. Patient A knows that he will have to take responsibility for reducing his hypertension, and Dr. Hypothetical wants to see if the patient really can do it. It would be far better to treat this case at Step Zero—diet, weight loss, exercise, and stress control—rather than putting Patient A on drugs, maybe for the rest of his life.

Patient A agrees to follow the diet given to him by the doctor, and also agrees to monitor his blood pressure at home. Dr. Hypothetical thinks that is fine, but he wants to use Patient A's cuff himself once or twice just to make sure it is accurate.

Dr. Hypothetical would not agree to home monitoring in all cases. Some patients are not emotionally equipped to handle knowing what their blood pressure is at every given moment. Some patients do not hear well enough to detect the gushing of blood through the artery, even with a powerful stethoscope. Some patients just are not smart enough to figure out how to work the cuff.

What Dr. Hypothetical wants is a good record of the blood pressure during Step Zero therapy. Not only will a record of readings indicate if the hypertension is excessively labile, it will demonstrate to the patient that diet, exercise, and weight loss really do bring about results.

When Patient A returns, Dr. Hypothetical will reevaluate results of blood pressure and weight loss. If, for example, the patient has lost ten points off the BP—getting it down to 150/90, and has also dropped ten pounds, then continued nondrug therapy might be considered.

But if there has been little or no progress, doctor and patient move to Step One.

Step One

Diuretics are drugs that promote secretion of salt in the urine and a higher output of urine. They are commonly used in classic Step One therapy.

In this case, Dr. Hypothetical puts his patient on diuretics. The patient is overweight and retains fluid, so diuretics seem the logical choice.

Had the patient presented symptoms suggesting other tendencies, such as a high tension level, Dr. Hypothetical might have chosen a drug called a *beta blocker* for Step One. A beta blocker slows the heart rate and lowers blood pressure by blocking certain nerve receptors. Diuretics have long been the drug of choice for Step One therapy; it has only been lately that beta blockers have been used as the first alternative.

In any event, Dr. Hypothetical has a wide choice of diuretics. He starts with a mild variety at a small dosage. One of the things he will do is to warn Patient A of the side effects.

"Don't take these pills right before you go to bed," he says, "because you'll be up all night going to the john. And don't take them right before a long car ride."

Once the patient and the doctor understand the goal of therapy, the patient will be sent home and another appointment will be made for two to four weeks from now—adequate time for the drug to take effect.

Ultimately, the physician wants the patient to be on as little medication as possible as long as the medication does the job. Some fine-tuning may have to be made in terms of drug or dosage. Drugs act differently on different bodies, and what might be too much for one patient will have little or no effect on another.

As a general rule of thumb, when more potent drugs are used the side effects are more potent. Some are actually dangerous, so it is a matter of balancing the risks versus the benefits.

Let's assume that Step One failed. Blood pressure was not reduced significantly by the diuretics.

Step Two

Drugs used in this level of therapy are mostly agents that block the *sympathetic* nervous system, the part of your nervous system that governs the fight-or-flight response. These include *beta blockers, alpha blockers,* and *sympatholytics.*

As we mentioned, beta blockers today are frequently used in Step One, although they can be used as a Step Two drug, depending on the physician's preference.

Beta blockers and alpha blockers do pretty much the same thing but in a different location. They both block *receptors:* The so-called beta receptors are located on organs such as the heart and kidneys, while the alpha receptors are in the muscle cells in the artery walls.

The discovery of receptors is a truly exciting breakthrough in pharmacology. In the past ten years or so, we have learned that a substance acts on a cell by attaching to a receptor—a biological term for a group of molecules that will receive only one specific type of chemical. Once the union is made between the substance and the receptor, a whole cascade of physiological events follow.

Beta blockers and alpha blockers, as the names imply, block this union at the receptors. The beta blockers interfere with the body signals that tell the heart to speed up. Alpha blockers interfere with the signal that instructs the arterioles to constrict. Beta and alpha blockers are sometimes lumped together in medical terminology and referred to as *adrenergic blockers* or *adrenergic inhibitors.* That is because the substance they are blocking is really adrenaline.

Sympatholytics are a different type of drug; they do not act on beta or alpha receptors but rather block the action of the sympathetic (fight-or-flight) nervous system as a whole. In times long past, this was done *surgically*—the sympathetic nervous system was cut in cases of runaway malignant hypertension.

Step Two drugs are, in general terms, more potent than Step One drugs. Dr. Hypothetical will make a diligent effort to list the more likely side effects of the drug he has prescribed, but there are literally a hundred *possible* side effects. If one should occur, he would like the patient to be aware that it may stem from the drug. For this reason, Dr. Hypothetical reminds his patient to ask the pharmacist to include the manufacturer's package insert when the prescription is filled for the first time. This insert is free, and although it is written in technical medical terms, it will help the patient become acquainted with adverse reactions sometimes associated with the medication.

As explained, Step Two medications can be highly potent and carry many side effects. Unfortunately, even these powerful preparations do not always reduce difficult hypertensions. If that is the case, a Step Three drug is added.

Step Three

This level of treatment usually involves use of *vasodilators*, drugs that dilate the arteries, opening them up. Arteries and arterioles have a muscular wall; when something goes wrong with the self-regulatory system, the muscular wall constricts and tightens the vessels. The tighter the vessel, of course, the greater the resistance and the higher the blood pressure.

These are very potent drugs and in general they carry a greater risk of unpleasant and/or dangerous side effects than do Step Two drugs. However, a physician deciding to go to Step Three feels that the benefit—controlling a dangerous case of hypertension—far outweighs the risk.

Sometimes, however, even vasodilators cannot do the job.

Step Four

While the other categories of drugs are indeed categories (meaning that they contain numbers of various medications), Step Four treatment means use of a specific drug called guanethedine. Guanethedine is a *ganglionic* blocker. A ganglion is a part of a nerve cell body that joins the nerve cell to an organ.

Guanethedine blocks the transmission of nerve impulses across the ganglia (plural of ganglion) very effectively, and does an excellent job of regulating out-of-control high blood pressure. However—and this is a big *however*—the cost of this is great because the ganglia also control such autonomic body functions as sexual activity, movement of food in the intestines, maintenance of blood supply to the brain when a person stands up quickly, and urination. Guanethedine can interfere with the normal functioning of these, and fainting upon arising must be watched carefully.

New Drugs Not Categorized in the Stepped Approach

One reason why the rigid application of the stepped approach is falling out of favor is the fact that newer drugs do not fit neatly into the steps. Two such drugs are *ACE inhibitors* and *calcium channel blockers*.

ACE, you may remember, is the angiotensin-converting enzyme. One increasingly popular such drug inhibits the whole renin–angiotensin I–angiotensin II–aldosterone cycle by preventing the conversion of angiotensin I into the problem-causing angiotensin II. Hence the term *ACE inhibitor*.

Calcium, you may also remember, acts at the cellular level to constrict arterioles. (This does not mean that eating calcium will cause high blood pressure or that not eating calcium will prevent it.) Calcium channel blockers keep calcium from entering the cell and therefore help prevent the constriction.

Since these medications are relatively new, there is no consensus among physicians on when to use them. But some physicians use the ACE inhibitors and calcium channel blockers as Step One, Step Two, or even Step Three medications.

The above steps are designed to treat the problem with the minimum amount of medication. A hypothetical patient may progress through all the steps when his or her doctor finds, for example, that each step just does not do enough to control the hypertension. When this system works, it spares—as much as possible—overmedication and the resulting side effects.

Stepped Care When It Doesn't Work

So what is wrong with the treatment described in the above category, "Stepped Care When It Works"? Nothing is intrinsically wrong with the approach—because in many cases it *does* work.

But things do not always work out so neatly, especially when doctors treat hypertension with a mechanical method that is not based on an accurate diagnosis. A volume-related problem might be treated with drugs that do not affect volume, or the reverse may happen.

In any event, treating the problem mechanically—without gaining a complete insight into the problem and the patient—may bring about an inadequate response to drug treatment, and as a consequence cause undesirable side effects. So if the treatment did not work because Dr. Hypothetical used the wrong key for the lock, he might compound matters by giving another inappropriate drug in addition to the first.

In the classic stepwise approach, drugs are added, so you may wind up with double the side effects. (This also works in the positive way, since some drugs may become considerably more potent when combined and attack the patient's problem more vigorously even though there are fewer drugs in the patient's system.)

One of the biggest problems with the strict application of the stepped approach is that it treats most hypertension as volume-related (too much fluid, therefore too much blood, therefore too much pressure). As stated a moment ago, a patient could very well be on two drugs—one of which is ineffective.

Modern treatment is based on greatly enhanced medical-chemical knowledge; it looks to the underlying problem as much as possible and tries to fit the key into the lock without fumbling with the wrong ones. A physician might find his patient a perfect candidate for an ACE inhibitor and skip the diuretics altogether. This avoids the expense, inconvenience, and possible dangers of unneeded drugs.

What This Means to a Hypertensive

So what does all this information have to do with you? For starters, it is likely that you may have had a bad experience in the past, and may have stopped taking your medication. Or possibly you are on medication now but do not like your treatment program. Maybe you just want more information and cannot get it from your doctor.

In any event, knowing why treatment works, and why it does not, is critically important to you because it is your hypertension and your responsibility. Treating hypertension is a lifelong process; your body will change and your blood pressure will change. The amount of drugs you are taking, or the types of drugs, may have to be changed.

Unless you take an active role in understanding and treating your hypertension, your treatments will not be as effective as they could be. And if you are not treating your hypertension—because of frustration with previous false starts or because you do not like the side effects of your medication—you are literally killing yourself inch by inch.

Hypertension treatment goes wrong in many ways. If you are unhappy with your treatment, get a second opinion. The information you are picking up in this book will help you elicit understandable recommendations from your doctor. Perhaps the course of your treatment is the best available and you will have to live with it. But possibly—just possibly—what you are getting is wrong for you.

Here are some cases in point:

- Craig is a highway patrolman. He does not take his diuretics any more because he just cannot get to a bathroom as frequently as he needs to. Craig's doctor, a rigid adherent to the diuretic as Step One approach, has told Craig he will just have to live with the problem.
- Sarah is a sixty-year-old woman who saw a doctor briefly five years ago and has not been back since. The medicine was relatively effective, but not particularly so. She could—if she expended the time and effort to resume regular medical care—be on a much more effective medicine with fewer side effects. She would be happier and healthier.
- Ellen is a thirty-four-year-old woman with a stoic disposition who does not even tell her doctor that she feels miserable because of the medicine. There are many other options she could try, but her doctor does not know of her problems because she keeps them to herself. As a result, Ellen is less than precise about taking her medicine.

The common thread is that better communication and more information can improve many less-than-perfect situations. It is often a case of trial and error, so never be reluctant to ask for new approaches to be tried if the old ones do not seem to be working.

Because drugs for hypertension are such an important part of the overall treatment program, they will be the subject of a comprehensive chapter—a chapter that may not provide exciting reading but will give you a handy reference source if you want to know more about the usage and possible side effects of a particular drug or drugs.

There are three points concerning all drug therapy that must be made now, though. They are extremely important and must not be overlooked.

1. *Never* go off an antihypertensive medication without talking to your doctor first. Some drugs can have dangerous effects if they are abruptly suspended.
2. *Never* slack off on taking your medication because you are "feeling better." As we have pointed out, hypertension usually produces no symptoms as it pounds away at your organs. By the time you notice symptoms, the damage may already be done and be irreversible.
3. Be wary of a scientific phenomenon called *tolerance*. An unscientific definition of tolerance is that a drug that you have been taking for a while is not now as potent because your body has grown "used to it." You may, in this case, need a higher dose or a new drug.

To Drug or Not to Drug?

A final consideration on the successes and failures of treatment concerns whether drugs should be involved at all. As mentioned earlier in the book, severe hypertension leaves no room for choice: It is either drugs or an early grave, and that is not a facetious statement.

But with mild or (in some cases) moderate hypertension, you and your physician have a choice. From the doctor's standpoint, he or she must evaluate whether you will make a sincere and immediate effort to modify diet, weight, and lifestyle.

Drug therapy is the easiest option for the doctor. If often involves nothing more than writing a prescription and doing a couple of follow-up checks. Drug-free therapy is the most difficult option for the physician because he or she must now assume the roles of dietician, physical education coach, and psychologist.

There is no question that drug-free therapy—using exercise, diet, and lifestyle changes—is the best choice for you, the patient. Lowering blood pressure through exercise, diet, and lifestyle changes is the best thing you can do for yourself *even if the results are not adequate and you still need drugs*. Here's why:

- In the event you can control hypertension without drugs, you have saved yourself from a lifetime of pill-taking.
- If you pay attention to Step Zero (drug free) therapy but still need drug treatment, you may need a lower dosage of the drug, sparing yourself side effects.
- If you pay attention to exercise, diet, and lifestyle, you may not need to advance to a more potent category of drugs, thus saving yourself more side effects and money.
- Being thin, cutting down on fatty foods, exercising, lowering salt intake, and coping better with stress cannot hurt you. Each factor will cut down your risks from other diseases as well as hypertension.

We will move on to address all the related topics in the next chapters. Drugs for hypertension are covered in the Chapter 3, followed by chapters on drug-free treatment in general, diet, exercise, and stress reduction.

First, some commonly asked questions concerning the topics covered in this chapter:

Q: Why do doctors add new drugs when progressing on the stepped approach, rather than discontinuing the less powerful drug and starting all over from scratch?

A: A good question, and a controversial one among physicians. Some doctors will eliminate the old drug; some keep adding. It depends on the individual situation. In some cases, the combination of two drugs works very well to attack a multifaceted hypertension problem.

Q: My doctor says drug-free therapy will just not work for me. Should I get a second opinion?

A: A second opinion will not hurt, but chances are your doctor has a very good reason for his or her opinion. Some cases of hypertension will just not respond to anything except pharmaceuticals.

Q: You mention that side effects of drugs are a major reason why treatment fails. Why do drugs for hypertension have so many side effects?

A: Because you are tinkering with a fantastically delicate mechanism and because we do not yet have all the answers about how that system works. We cannot design drugs totally free from unwanted effects.

But because of the greater selection of drugs available today—as opposed to even five years ago—you have a much better chance of avoiding significant side effects. Often, substances do not affect all people the same way. Coffee, or shellfish, or rich desserts bother some people but not others. It is the same with drugs. If a drug produces too many side effects, you and your doctor may be able to find a drug that has the same good points but fewer or different bad points.

[3]
What You Should Know
about Drugs for
Hypertension

This chapter is technically out of order, we suppose, because drug treatments are often considered after the possibility of drug-free therapy is evaluated. Drug-free control of hypertension is the subject of the following four chapters.

However, the information presented here is a direct expansion of the material presented in the discussion of stepped care, and directly relates to the body's workings as described in Chapter 1. Also, because you are reading this book in the first place, it is likely that you are now taking antihypertensive medication, and would like some understanding of those medications before considering ways that may enable you to reduce your dosage or eliminate those drugs.

So, let's look at medications for treating high blood pressure. You remember from the last chapter that the stepped care approach usually looks something like this:

1. Step One
   a. diuretics
   b. beta blockers (sometimes, although beta blockers are frequently thought of as Step Two drugs)
2. Step Two
   a. adrenergic blocking agents—meaning alpha blockers and beta blockers (remember, beta blockers are used in Step One or Step Two)
   b. sympatholytics
3. Step Three
   a. vasodilators
4. Step Four
   a. guanethedine
5. New Drugs Not Yet Categorized in Stepped Approach
   a. ACE inhibitors
   b. calcium channel blockers

Depending on your personal degree of hypertension, you may, through your lifetime, take none of the above or, conceivably, all of the above. It is important to have some basic knowledge about the effects of these medications and the side effects. By understanding what these substances do to your internal system of valves and switches, you can take a more active role in lifelong hypertension control. At the very least, you will have a reassuring understanding of why these drugs produce their particular effects and side effects.

So, let's examine each category of drugs in the order listed above.

Diuretics

A diuretic causes *diuresis*, which means water extraction as well as salt removal. The goal of taking a diuretic is to reduce the volume of plasma (the liquid portion of blood) in the body. The removal of salt in turn causes more depletion of liquid. These are the oldest of all antihypertensive agents and in terms of prescriptions written daily are almost certainly the most extensively used.

Modern diuretics fall into three basic categories, depending on their site of action: *thiazide*, *loop*, and *potassium-sparing*.

Thiazide Diuretics

These drugs were developed from the old sulfa compounds used before the advent of modern antibiotics. Thiazide had limited value as an infection fighter, but researchers found that it did a marvelous job of diuresis. In addition, thiazide diuretics combine well with other *hypotensive* drugs (another name for drugs used to lower blood pressure) and increase the effect of other drugs.

A well-known thiazide diuretic is chlorothiazide, marketed under trade names including Diuril. (The term *chlorothiazide* is the chemical name, what we often call the generic name; the trade name is the name invented by the drug company when it sells that drug under its own brand. Generic names are not capitalized, but trade names are. The generic versus trade name question will be discussed in more detail later in the chapter.)

Thiazide diuretics are relatively mild and their effect lasts a long time. Thiazides act directly on the kidneys to bring about diuresis.

Loop Diuretics

Loop diuretics accomplish the same goal as thiazide diuretics but they work on a "looped" portion of the kidneys' filtration system. Because of their different site of action, loop diuretics are considerably more potent. They can produce a very rapid formation of urine and can also produce considerable inconvenience, especially for someone who cannot get to a bathroom frequently.

Loop diuretics are prescribed for patients with a large amount of excess fluid that the physician wants depleted quickly. These drugs are also quite useful for patients who have concomitant disease such as congestive heart failure.

The compound furosemide, marketed under the trade name Lasix, is a frequently used loop diuretic.

Potassium-Sparing Diuretics

One problem with diuretics is that they wash the chemical known as potassium out of the body. If you do not take in enough potassium to begin with, or if your body is particularly susceptible to potassium washout, you can experience side effects such as weakness, lethargy, and muscle spasm. More serious, and more rare, side effects include heartbeat irregularities.

Potassium-sparing diuretics are useful for people subject to side effects from potassium loss, but the drugs are very expensive in general and are not as potent as loop diuretics.

Sprironolactone (Aldactone)—we will often be giving the chemical name, followed by brand name in parentheses, the standard method for this type of double notation—is a common potassium-sparing diuretic. The drug spironolactone is not without its problems, though. One is breast enlargement, a side effect not at all popular with men who take the drug.

Some drug companies have combined the categories of diuretics into one agent that magnifies the good qualities of both. A good example is the drug called Dyazide. Ask your physician about the possibility of using such a drug if you are experiencing quite a bit of difficulty with your diuretic.

Adrenergic Blockers

As you may remember from last chapter's discussion, these agents block the hormone adrenaline, keeping it from forming a union at beta and alpha receptors. Both the beta blockers and the alpha blockers prevent the hormone from transmitting a message—a message from the out-of-kilter blood pressure control mechanism.

Beta Blockers

These drugs inhibit the beta receptors, which are found in smooth muscle cells in the heart and lung. In general, they cause a lowering of blood pressure by making the heart pump less effectively and decreasing the force with which it pumps. They probably have an effect in the kidneys, but we do not know for sure.

There are two types of beta receptors, beta one and beta two. It is not important to delve further into the anatomy of beta reception, but it is worthwhile for you to know that when beta two receptors are blocked, the bronchial tubes may be narrowed, making beta two blocking drugs a poor choice for anyone with asthma. This is an example of why your doctor will do a comprehensive history and examination before prescribing an antihypertensive drug.

Propranolol (Inderal) is the prototype beta blocker. It has been in existence for twenty years and is still the most widely used beta blocking agent.

Side effects of beta blockers in general include a slowing of the heartbeat, fatigue, and sleep disorders including insomnia and bizarre dreams (though not necessarily nightmares).

Alpha Blockers

The alpha receptors are located in the arterial system. It is thought that alpha blockers lower blood pressure by causing dilation of the medium-sized arteries. While this does reduce blood pressure, it also causes problems with too-rapid a blood pressure drop when the patient stands up quickly. Known as *postural hypotension*, this effect can result in dizziness, especially after the first dose of the drug is taken.

What is postural hypotension? When someone with a normally performing nervous system stands up abruptly, the nervous system sends out frantic signals to keep the blood pressure the same or slightly elevated; the reason, of course, is that blood flow to the brain must be maintained. But when the nervous system is blunted by a blocker, the signals may not make it in time and dizziness or fainting may occur. A doctor must always warn patients about this side effect. Injuries caused by postural hypotension frequently occur when someone is awakened by a call and jumps out of bed to get the phone. Therefore, extra care is warranted when taking the first dose of an alpha blocker.

Other side effects may include heart palpitations, lethargy, and headaches. Depression and impotence sometimes occur.

New alpha blockers are being developed and will probably be available soon.

Prazosin (Minipress) is the most widely used alpha blocker.

Sympatholytics

Use of this type of drug inhibits the sympathetic nervous system and causes a lowering of blood pressure. The sympathetic nervous system governs your fight-or-flight responses.

Two of the earliest drugs produced in this category are clonidine (Catapres) and methyldopa (Aldomet). Clonidine has a powerful effect in the brain and as a result can also produce sedation. Methyldopa sometimes causes a type of anemia and can induce hepatitis, probably as an allergic reaction to the drug. Both drugs can interfere with sexual function.

The most serious side effect of both of these agents is postural hypotension.

Incidentally, methyldopa and clonidine are sometimes referred to as *central adrenergic inhibitors*. This category of drugs can act either centrally, meaning in the brain, or peripherally, meaning outside of the brain. A common peripherally acting sympatholitic (translation: a drug that affects the sympathetic nervous system but does not do its work in the brain) is reserpine.

Reserpine is one of the oldest of antihypertensive medications. It is derived from a plant called *Rauwolfia serpentina*. The root of the rauwolfia plant was an ancient remedy used in India for treatment of the insane. Its tranquilizing effects were later found to lower blood pressure as well. Essentially, reserpine reduces cardiac output and the resistance of the blood vessels (peripheral resistance).

Reserpine is one of the cheapest antihypertensive medications available but it can sometimes produce disabling depression, particularly among senior citizens.

Vasodilators

These drugs open up the arterioles, relaxing the constriction present in many hypertension cases, and causing decreased resistance to blood flow and a lowering of BP.

Two of the most common vasodilators in use today are hydralazine (Apresoline) and minoxidil (Loniten). These are very potent drugs. Unfortunately, they can cause changes in heart function and can even lead to heart attack. Because of this, minoxidil, the stronger of the two, is generally used with a beta blocker to slow heart rate.

(What happens is that the nervous system senses a drop in blood pressure because of the dilation of the arterioles. The heart is signaled to start pumping faster; the phenomenon—called a reflex tachycardia— is slowed by the beta blocker, which blocks the heart's receipt of the nervous system's frantic signal for more blood.)

To give you an idea of the complexity of prescribing vasodilators, consider the fact that the physician will generally also prescribe a diuretic. Why? Because as blood pressure falls due to vasodilation, the body responds not only by increasing the heart rate but by retaining fluid. Therefore, a patient on powerful vasodilators could swell up with a thirty- to forty-pound weight gain without the diuretic. Because of this complex web of reactions, vasodilators are typically not used as *monotherapy* (used alone) for treatment of hypertension.

This is one example of how intricate the body's feedback systems are, and why an agent that blocks one step might cause the body to overreact and produce a complication as severe as the original problem. Such interactions also show why the physician sometimes does not eliminate previously used drugs when adding another drug.

Minoxidil also causes stimulation of hair growth for reasons not yet understood.

Guanethedine

By its very nature, this is a drug of last resort, used only for severe cases of hypertension. It causes depletion of a hormone called norepinephrine—a close relative of adrenaline—at the nerve endings. It can have significant side effects, including postural hypotension, severe sexual dysfunction, ejaculation backward into the urinary bladder, and a slowing of the heartbeat.

It is not generally used in monotherapy; a diuretic is often added.

Two of the most promising developments in modern pharmacology are ACE inhibitors and calcium channel blockers. They are used at various levels in the stepped care system.

ACE Inhibitors

Medications such as captopril (Capoten) and enalapril (Vasotec) are good examples of how modern drugs fit the lock-and-key approach.

Captopril is a promising new antihypertensive agent that was initially developed in Europe. It is by far the most specific of antihypertensive agents. Captopril inhibits the chain of chemical reactions that eventually cause vascular constriction and sodium retention. It is extremely effective for kidney-related hypertension problems. This medication—derived from snake venom—is used on a two- or three-times-a-day regimen.

Captopril has been used in the stepped system at anywhere from Step Two to Step Four. Its side effects include a reduction of white blood cells in the blood and release of protein in the urine.

Enalapril (Vasotec) is another exciting development in this field. It can be given on a once-a-day regimen and effectively lowers blood pressure for a twenty-four-hour period.

Calcium Channel Blockers

These drugs, also called calcium entry blockers, were originally developed for treating angina. As discussed in the previous chapter, they inhibit calcium entry into cells.

Calcium channel blockers are perfect for the elderly patient who suffers from both angina and hypertension (which often go hand in hand). We are not quite sure as to the exact mechanism by which calcium channel blockers reduce blood pressure.

These are relatively powerful agents and could be used as Step Two or Step Three drugs. Because of their profound effect on the heart, they can carry side effects such as abnormal slowing of heartbeat, and they may even aggravate congestive heart failure by inhibiting the pumping mechanism of the heart.

At this writing, there were three calcium entry blockers available in the United States: diltiazem (Cardizem), nifedipine (Procardia), and verapamil (Calan and Isoptin). It is likely that there will be many more available in coming years.

Deciding on a Drug

So how does a physician sort through the many drugs available and determine which one you will be taking? A number of factors are involved, including the severity of your hypertension, the peculiarities of your particular case, your general physical condition, and the doctor's assessment of how strictly you will stay on your program.

Again, remember that there is a certain amount of trial and error involved. One drug may prove ineffective. A particular medication may cause unpleasant side effects; a change to another may control your hypertension with minimal or no side effects.

It is a complicated affair. Here are some examples of how the process works.

CASE HISTORY 1

PATIENT: Seventy-year-old woman. History of angina, history of obesity. Fluid retention with mild congestive heart failure. BP is 160/110.

Some end-organ damage noted during physical. Significant volume retention noted.

BP is probably more volume dependent, but vasoconstriction is a factor.

PRESCRIPTION: Furosemide, a powerful loop diuretic. Thiazide diuretic probably would be too weak to do the job, and this woman needs fluid reduced quickly.

PROGNOSIS: Patient will be seen weekly for BP and weight loss monitoring. If furosemide does not bring BP under control, methyldopa will be tried because of methyldopa's gentleness on the heart.

CASE HISTORY 2

PATIENT: Nineteen-year-old male college athlete. Has had hypertension for about three years. Very active in sports, sexually active. BP last read at 150/90. Patient is not overweight, does not eat highly salted foods, does not smoke.

PRESCRIPTION: Propranolol. Patient is concerned about effect on sexual performance and athletic performance. Possibility that he would not comply with treatment if such side effects occurred. Propranolol chosen because beta blockers very rarely cause sexual dysfunction (as diuretics sometimes do) and will not affect patient's alertness on practice field.

PROGNOSIS: Good chance of compliance with drug therapy because patient specified his particular needs.

CASE HISTORY 3

PATIENT: Forty-five-year-old male, office manager, under extreme time pressure at work. Recently divorced, heavy drinker and smoker. Presented with BP of 150/98.

PRESCRIPTION: Step Zero is worth a try; weight loss, cessation of smoking, and reduction of drinking may be effective, as it appears much of patient's hypertension is induced by those factors. Stress also appears to be major factor; referral to psychologist for stress reduction therapy indicated.

PROGNOSIS: Patient seems intelligent and motivated to lower BP without drugs. If he continues to have significantly elevated blood pressure, clonidine may be drug of choice because of minimal side effects and because of new skin patch method of dispensing. (Clonidine can be released through the skin from a patch applied to the skin once a week; see Chapter 9 for details.) Patient is often tied up in meetings and says he can not take pills on precise schedule.

Writing the Prescription

Once your doctor has determined which drug to use, how does he or she determine the amount? In general, the amounts are pretty standard, but allowances will be made for very large or very small people. Keep in mind that the doctor almost always will start low and work up; many physicians also will start with the cheapest drug and work up to more expensive drugs if they are needed.

Expense is a factor you and your doctor should consider. Some medicines for hypertension are quite expensive. A drug that costs $30 a month costs $360 a year, and over a lifetime these costs will really add up; some drugs are significantly more expensive than the example just given.

Your physician may or may not write a prescription for the generic (chemical) name of the drug and leave it up to the pharmacist to fill the prescription with the cheapest generic. A doctor may also have the option of indicating on the prescription whether a generic substitute may be made for the trade name specified.

In fairness, there are two sides to the generic situation. Usually, a generic drug is cheaper, but some generics have been proven to be not as effective as the brand-name drugs. Essentially, this is a question you and your doctor will have to sort out for yourselves.

The chart on the following pages will give you some insight into the various drugs used for treatment of hypertension. It has been reprinted with permission from *Patient Care* magazine; the column relating to side effects and precautions has been adapted by the authors because the original remarks were in technical medical terminology.

When reading this chart, you will first look to the category of the drug for which you want more information. The categories are:

Diuretics
  I. Thiazides and related sulfonamide diuretics
 II. Loop diuretics
III. Potassium-sparing agents

Antihypertensive drugs used in monotherapy

The following drugs may be used in initial therapy for hypertension. Combination drugs and those not used alone as initial agents have not been listed. Unless otherwise indicated, the dosages represent a once-a-day schedule.

Generic and trade names	Dosages (mg/d)*		Average wholesale price** (per 100 tablets)		Comments
	Initial	Maximum	At initial dosage	At maximum dosage	
DIURETICS					
I. Thiazides and related sulfonamide diuretics					All thiazides and related sulfonamide diuretics:
Bendroflumethiazide (Naturetin)	2.5	5.0	$18.53	$29.18	—may produce lowered potassium levels in blood, resulting in weakness, lethargy, and muscle spasms. More severe reactions include irregular heartbeats and the risk of death in extreme cases.
Benzthiazide (Aquatag)	25	50	***	11.40	—may produce high levels of calcium, sugar, fats (cholesterol and triglycerides), and uric acid (which may cause gout) in the blood.
(Exna)	25	50	***	11.10	—can cause sexual impotency.
Chlorothiazide (Diuril)	250	500	6.56	10.40	—work by increasing the amount and frequency of urination.
Chlorthalidone (Hygroton)	25	50-100	21.15	26.08 (50-mg tablets)	—do not work well for patients with bad kidneys.
(Thalitone)	25	50-100	14.16	***	The physician should draw blood periodically to check potassium, calcium, sugar, fat, and uric acid levels.
Cyclothiazide (Anhydron)	1	2	***	17.20	
(Fluidil)	1	2	***	(Not listed)	

*Some dosages differ from what is recommended in the *Physicians' Desk Reference* and the manufacturer's package insert. The maximum suggested dosage may be exceeded in resistant cases.
**Based on information in *The Drug Topics Red Book,* Oradell, NJ, Medical Economics Co, Inc, 1985. Unless otherwise indicated, the price is that of 100 tablets or capsules in the strength of the recommended dosage.
***Not available in strength of recommended dosage.

This drug chart has been developed with the aid of our roundtable panelists and with information adapted from Tables 5 and 6 in *The 1984 Report of the Joint National Committee on Detection, Evaluation, and Treatment of High Blood Pressure,* US Dept of Health and Human Services, Public Health Service, National Institutes of Health (NIH Publication No 84-1088), 1984, pp 18, 20-1. *continued*
This chart is reproduced here with permission from *Patient Care,* November 30, 1985. Copyright © 1985, Patient Care Communications, Inc., Darien, CT. All rights reserved. The column headed "Comments" has been adapted by the authors, with permission, from the chart's original columns "Side effects" and "Precautions."

67

Antihypertensive drugs used in monotherapy continued

Generic and trade names	Dosages (mg/d)*		Average wholesale price** (per 100 tablets)		Comments
	Initial	Maximum	At initial dosage	At maximum dosage	
DIURETICS continued					
I. Thiazides and related sulfonamide diuretics continued					
Hydrochlorothiazide (Esidrix)	12.5-25.0	50	$6.32 (25-mg tablets)	$10.00	
(HydroDIURIL)	12.5-25.0	50	6.56 (25-mg tablets)	10.40	
(Oretic)	12.5-25.0	50	4.04 (25-mg tablets)	6.39	
Hydroflumethiazide (Diucardin)	25	50	***	10.63	
(Saluron)	25	50	***	21.00	
Indapamide (Lozol)	2.5	5.0	31.73	***	
Methyclothiazide (Aquatensen)	2.5	5.0	***	21.67	
(Enduron)	2.5	5.0	12.20	16.13	
Metolazone (Diulo)	2.5	10.0	13.25	19.61	
(Zaroxolyn)	2.5	10.0	15.35	20.87	
Polythiazide (Renese)	2	4	22.90	38.28	

Drug					
Quinethazone (Hydromox)	50	100	37.73	•••	
Trichlormethiazide (Metahydrin)	2	4	13.50	21.52	
(Naqua)	2	4	15.60	24.24	
II. Loop diuretics					All **loop diuretics** can cause basically the same side effects as the thiazides listed above. In addition, all loop diuretics listed here: —may produce low sodium (salt) levels in the elderly. —can work in patients with bad kidneys.
Bumetanide† (Bumex)	0.25 bid	5.00 bid	11.22 (0.5-mg tablets)	15.78 (1.0-mg tablets)	
Ethacrynic acid† (Edecrin)	25 bid	100 bid	14.74	21.01 (50-mg tablets)	
Furosemide (Lasix)	40 bid	240 bid	12.45	20.60 (80-mg tablets)	
III. Potassium-sparing agents					All **potassium-sparing agents** may cause a build-up of too much potassium, especially in patients with bad kidneys. **Spironolactone** may cause sexual impotency, breast enlargement, and breast pain. **Trimaterene** may cause stomach and intestinal problems.
Amiloride HCl (Midamor)	5	10	22.44	•••	
Spironolactone (Aldactone)	50	100	38.30	64.21	
Triamterene (Dyrenium)	50	100	13.80	17.30	

*Some dosages differ from what is recommended in the *Physicians' Desk Reference* and the manufacturer's package insert. The maximum suggested dosage may be exceeded in resistant cases.
**Based on information in *The Drug Topics Red Book*, Oradell, NJ, Medical Economics Co. Inc., 1985. Unless otherwise indicated, the price is that of 100 tablets or capsules in the strength of the recommended dosage.
***Not available in strength of recommended dosage.
†Hypertension is not an FDA-recognized indication for this drug.

Antihypertensive drugs used in monotherapy continued

Generic and trade names	Dosages (mg/dj)*		Average wholesale price** (per 100 tablets)		Comments
	Initial	Maximum	At initial dosage	At maximum dosage	
ADRENERGIC INHIBITORS					
I. β-Adrenergic blockers					All beta blockers: —should never be stopped abruptly, since heart rate and blood pressure may go up rapidly. —may cause a slow heart rate, tiredness, inability to sleep, bizarre dreams, sexual dysfunction (rare), and high triglycerides in blood. —should be used with care in patients with asthma, heart failure, diabetes, or severe hardening of the arteries. Acebutolol HCl, atenolol, and metoprolol tartrate work on the heart in low doses.
Acebutolol HCl (Sectral)	200	400 bid	$29.76	$39.56	
Atenolol (Tenormin)	25-50	100	39.86 (50-mg tablets)	59.77	
Metoprolol tartrate (Lopressor)	25-50 bid	150-200 bid	19.20 (50-mg tablets)	34.55 (100-mg tablets)	
Nadolol (Corgard)	20-40	80-160	41.81 (40-mg tablets)	56.10 (80-mg tablets) 81.18 (160-mg tablets)	
Pindolol (Visken)	10 bid	30 bid	29.88	***	
Propranolol HCl (Inderal)	10-40 bid	160-240 bid	9.64 (10-mg tablets) 19.51 (40-mg tablets)	32.53 (80-mg tablets)	

70

	80	480	36.42	59.11 (160-mg capsules)	
(Inderal LA)					
Timolol maleate (Blocadren)	5-10 bid	20-30 bid	21.13 (5-mg tablets) 26.13 (10-mg tablets)	48.19 (20-mg tablets)	All **central adrenergic inhibitors** may cause dry mouth, drowziness, tiredness, sexual impotency, forgetfulness, and confusion.
II. Central adrenergic inhibitors					
Clonidine HCl (Catapres)	0.05-0.10 bid	0.6 bid	19.83 (0.1-mg tablets)	38.07 (0.3-mg tablets)	**Clonidine HCl** and **guanabenz acetate** may cause elevations in blood pressure if stopped suddenly.
Guanabenz acetate (Wytensin)	4 bid	16 bid	23.31 (4-mg tablets)	35.00 (8-mg tablets)	**Methyldopa** may cause a low red-cell count (anemia) and liver inflammation (a kind of chemical hepatitis).
Methyldopa (Aldomet)	250 bid	1,000 bid	19.11 (250-mg tablets)	34.91 (500-mg tablets)	
III. Peripheral adrenergic antagonist					This agent may cause sexual impotency; also, nasal congestion (similar to sinusitis).
Reserpine	0.1	0.5	3.14	5.31 (0.25-mg tablets)	**Reserpine** may cause tiredness; it should not be used for anyone with history or symptoms suggesting depression.
IV. α-Adrenergic blocker					
Prazosin HCl (Minipress)	1 bid or tid	10 bid or tid	18.70 (1-mg capsules)	43.78 (5-mg capsules)	**Alpha blockers** may cause fainting after the first dose, postural hypotension, dizziness, palpitations, or weakness. These are used with caution in elderly patients.

*Some dosages differ from what is recommended in the *Physicians' Desk Reference* and the manufacturer's package insert. The maximum suggested dosage may be exceeded in resistant cases.

**Based on information in *The Drug Topics Red Book*, Oradell, NJ, Medical Economics Co, Inc, 1985. Unless otherwise indicated, the price is that of 100 tablets or capsules in the strength of the recommended dosage.

***Not available in strength of recommended dosage.

Antihypertensive drugs used in monotherapy continued

Generic and trade names	Dosages (mg/d)*		Average wholesale price** (per 100 tablets)		Comments
	Initial	Maximum	At initial dosage	At maximum dosage	
ADRENERGIC INHIBITORS continued					
V. Combined α- and β-adrenergic blocker					Agents in this category may cause a slow heart rate. They should be used with care in patients with asthma, heart failure, diabetes, or severe hardening of the arteries.
Labetalol HCl (Normodyne)	100-200 bid	600 bid	$23.40 (200-mg tablets)	$31.14 (300-mg tablets)	
(Trandate)	100-200 bid	600 bid	23.40 (200-mg tablets)	31.14 (300-mg tablets)	
ANGIOTENSIN-CONVERTING ENZYME (ACE) INHIBITOR					
Captopril (Capoten)	25 bid	50 tid	30.73	50.75	Captopril may cause a rash or abnormal taste in the mouth. It also may cause kidney failure in special cases, and may cause protein in the urine.
CALCIUM ENTRY BLOCKERS					All **calcium entry (channel) blockers** may cause headache, severe low blood pressure, and constipation, and may increase levels of the drug digoxin in the blood.
Diltiazem HCl* (Cardizem)	30 qid	60 qid	21.88	35.63	**Diltiazem HCl** may cause nausea and should be used with caution in patients with weak hearts.
Nifedipine* (Procardia)	10 tid	60 tid	27.31	†	**Nifedipine** may cause a rapid heartbeat and worsen angina; may cause flushing and fluid retention.
Verapamil HCl* (Calan)	80 tid	120 qid	24.24	32.78	**Verapamil HCl** may cause a slow heart rate, flushing, and fluid retention.
(Isoptin)	80 tid	120 qid	22.03	†	

*Some dosages differ from what is recommended in the *Physicians' Desk Reference* and the manufacturer's package insert. The maximum suggested dosage may be exceeded in resistant cases.
**Based on information in *The Drug Topics Red Book*, Oradell, NJ, Medical Economics Co, Inc, 1985. Unless otherwise indicated, the price is that of 100 tablets or capsules in the strength of the recommended dosage.
***Hypertension is not an FDA-recognized indication for this drug.
†Not available in strength of recommended dosage.

Adrenergic Inhibitors

I. Beta blockers (On the chart, these are listed as β-adrenergic blockers; that symbol is the Greek letter beta.)

II. Central adrenergic inhibitors (what we called sympatholytics in the earlier discussion)

III. Peripheral adrenergic antagonist (This is reserpine; as explained earlier, reserpine is a sympatholytic also called a peripheral adrenergic antagonist because of its site of action.)

IV. Alpha blocker (shown on the chart as α-adrenergic blocker)

V. Combined (A drug that works on both alpha and beta receptors is listed.)

Angiotensin-Converting Enzyme (ACE) Inhibitor

Calcium Entry Blockers (the same as calcium channel blockers; only the name is different)

The generic names of the drugs are in boldface and listed on top. The trade names are below in parentheses.

The dosages are listed in milligrams per day. There are some abbreviations you will need to know to read the chart:

bid: Twice a day, usually at twelve-hour intervals
tid: Three times a day, usually at eight-hour intervals
qid: Four times a day, usually at six-hour intervals

The chart also lists average wholesale price per hundred tablets. Prices, of course, can and will change after this book is printed, but you still can use the price listings as a tool for comparison. If you are on an expensive drug, for example, you can at least ask your doctor if a less expensive drug that appears on the chart would be appropriate for you.

In the last column, we have listed some of the major side effects, precautions, and special considerations you should know about.

Note that this chart gives information on drugs used in monotherapy—that is, used alone. The fact that vasodilators and the ganglion blocker are not used as monotherapy accounts for their absence. We have added information on these categories of drugs, as follows:

Vasodilators

In general, vasodilators may cause a rapid heart rate and worsen angina, and should be used in conjunction with a beta blocker.

Hydralazine (Apresoline) is usually prescribed in minimum dosages of 25–50 mg bid and maximum dosages of 100 mg bid. The average wholesale price for 25-mg tablets is $11.27 per hundred. Hydralazine (Apresoline) may cause headaches, nausea, and tiredness. It may also cause serious "lupus" syndrome (which is the body reacting against itself), causing pain and inflammation.

Minoxidil (Loniten) is usually prescribed in minimum doses of 2.5–5 mg bid and maximum doses of 20 mg bid. The average wholesale price for 2.5-mg tablets is $21.32 per hundred. This agent may cause water retention and hair growth. It should be used with a beta blocker and a diuretic. It can be a potent agent for lowering blood pressure.

Ganglion Blocker

Guanethedine (Ismelin) is generally prescribed in minimum dosages of 10 mg qid and maximum dosages of 150 mg qid. The average wholesale price of the lower dosage is $24.68 for a hundred tablets.

This drug may cause postural hypotension made worse by exercise, hot weather, and alcohol consumption. It may cause diarrhea, decreased sex drive, water retention, or slow heart rate. Some antidepressant drugs (tricyclics) may interfere with its effect.

Guanethedine (Ismelin) should not be used with over-the-counter cold preparations because they can cause severe increase in blood pressure.

As mentioned earlier, if hypertension can be controlled without using drugs, it is always to your advantage. We will discuss some possible options in the next portion of the book. First, though, some common questions on the material covered so far:

Q: I have heard that once you get on drug treatment for hypertension, your body is addicted and you can never get off drugs. Is that true?

A: No, there is no truth in that. In some cases a drug can cause withdrawal symptoms, but it does not mean that by the act of taking antihypertensive drugs you have precluded drug-free control.

Q: Why aren't tranquilizers used to lower high blood pressure?

A: In some cases—especially where stress is a major factor—some tranquilization is used. In fact, some hypotensive medications have a tranquilizing effect. However, simple tranquilization is not as effective as specific hypotensive medication in lowering blood pressure.

Q: There are so many side effects. Am I doomed to being miserable because I have to take medicine for hypertension?

A: No. Many medications, especially newer ones, provide maximum lowering of blood pressure with a minimum of side effects. But since many people do suffer side effects in various degrees (ranging from simply noticing the drug to becoming ill), side effects are an important point to consider.

Note that many side effects will lessen or disappear after you take the drug for a while. Nausea, in particular, is usually a symptom of the body's *initial* reaction to the drug; as the body adjusts, the nausea usually will not reoccur.

[4]
Drug-Free
Treatments

As we have seen, antihypertensive medications are wonderful agents—indeed, they are every bit as life-saving as antibiotics. They are not, however, without problems. Chemists and biologists simply cannot tinker with the human metabolism without some unexpected and unwanted results, at least not yet. And while most patients can take antihypertensive medications without significant side effects, all of them would be better off if they did not have to take medications in the first place.

Some hypertensives can make changes in their lifestyle to reduce the amount of medication they take or to get off medication altogether. If you can control your blood pressure without drugs, you are *always* ahead of the game. Why? There are four major reasons:

1. *Greater safety.* Most nonpharmacological methods of blood pressure control have few if any adverse side effects. The benefit-to-risk ratio of losing weight, for instance, is very good. There is some risk of injury or illness involved in physical fitness—you could break a leg or have a heart attack—but in most cases the risk is very small in comparison to the benefit. You have absolutely nothing to lose by trying to control stress.

2. *Lower cost.* Many antihypertensive drugs are quite costly, whereas diet, fitness, and stress reduction are inexpensive and can actually reduce some of the other medical and food costs you incur.

3. *Avoidance of drug interaction.* Some drugs lower blood pressure but may lead to other things you are trying to avoid, such as elevations in blood fat and blood sugar levels.

4. *Reduction of other risk factors.* Step Zero treatment is aimed at controlling hypertension, but can also improve your health in general. Exercise and weight loss will certainly help your heart and will probably cut down on blood fat (lipid) levels.

It is clear that Step Zero treatment—the nondrug approach to controlling hypertension—is the way to go if at all possible.

Who Can Benefit from Step Zero Treatment?

Theoretically, everyone. In practice, the answer is tied to the type of hypertension you have. We feel that a majority of mild hypertensives—probably 70 to 75 percent—could eliminate the need for drug treatment by diet, exercise, and stress control. Approximately 40 to 50 percent of moderate hypertensives could probably do the same.

For the rest of the mild and moderates and all of the severes, it is pretty clear that drug therapy is essential.

Wait a minute! Don't flip the page because you think you are ruled out of Step Zero therapy, because you absolutely are not—even if you are among those mild or moderates who will always need medication or if you are a severe. Step Zero can help reduce the quantity and potency of your medications, lower the resulting side effects and metabolic imbalances, and improve the overall functioning of all your other body systems.

Your doctor will make the final decision on whether you can go drug free or can incorporate Step Zero with drug therapy. The first judgment tool for determining the course of Step Zero is always a complete physical; this is the only way your physican can assess your chances for success.

If you already have organ damage, perhaps the result of a previous stroke or coronary artery disease, you can still benefit from drug-free therapy, but you will need medical supervision to do it. And if your hypertension is in the moderate to severe range and is coupled with the existing organ damage, this almost always indicates the need for pharmacological treatment in addition to good diet, exercise, and stress control.

In addition, we recommend that those who have organ damage, and anyone over forty who presents evidence of organ damage, particularly heart disease, should have an exercise stress text, a measurement of how the body responds to vigorous activity. The exercise stress test—

done on a treadmill—is a successful, sensitive, and accurate way to determine just how much exercise you should be doing.

Another benefit of a stress test is that it often allows doctors to evaluate the effect of exercise on blood pressure. Sometimes, a blood pressure may make a significant potentially damaging rise with exercise.

Other associated risk factors that often warrant a stress test include diabetes, high cholesterol, smoking, obesity, excess alcohol consumption, and a strong family history of heart disease.

The Effects of Step Zero Treatment

New studies and data are uncovering some of the benefits of diet, exercise, and stress reduction in the prevention of hypertension and the management of hypertension. While studies and statistical data are not always conclusive—nor can they be conclusive, given the current state of our knowledge of the body—a prudent and informed health professional will generally conclude that:

1. By far the most effective Step Zero method of fighting hypertension is maintaining a normal body weight. Keep your weight within 20 percent of the so-called ideal weights listed in Chapter 5. If you maintain a good body weight, there is strong evidence that you can reduce hypertension, prevent it from developing, or at least forestall its onset.
2. Reducing salt is often—but not always—effective in lowering BP. *Increasing* your intake of calcium and potassium would appear to be helpful, although the evidence for calcium and potassium action is far from conclusive.
3. Exercise probably will lower blood pressure, and is a factor in keeping other related body systems in good working order.
4. Stress reduction will also probably lower blood pressure, although the odds are not as great as with items 1, 2, and 3. Stress control also appears to work in other ways to preserve health, and it definitely makes your short stay on this planet more pleasant.
5. Other factors influence BP to varying degrees. Smoking is important. The dangers have been so well documented that there

is little point in pursuing the issue other than to point out that cigarettes do their damage on virtually all levels of the cardiovascular system. Reduction of alcohol and caffeine probably can help reduce blood pressure.

You have probably noticed that these conclusions are couched in the language of science—that is, it "appears," and this "probably" causes that to happen. As explained in Chapter One, studies and statistics are not always conclusive; at various points in the following chapters on diet, exercise, and stress reduction we will point out what the evidence says and what it does not say.

But in general terms, and to the best of our ability, we have found the above conclusions to be accurate. For all practical purposes, we *know* that Step Zero treatment *can* lower blood pressure. Results will differ from patient to patient but you can probably—there is that word again—use a conscientious program of diet, exercise, and stress reduction to lower your systolic BP by 10 to 15 points and your diastolic BP by 5 to 10 points. Greater reductions are possible, and there are many additional benefits to be gained from a fit body and mind.

How to Start

Tell your doctor you sincerely want to give Step Zero a try. Unless there is some compelling complication specific to your case, it is hard to believe that there is a doctor in the world who would not at least consider the idea.

Practically speaking, what a doctor usually would do in this case is to put you on a salt-reduction and weight-loss diet, make sure you are following it, and periodically and slowly decrease the amount of medication once you are making gains on your Step Zero program.

If blood pressure goes down and stays down, your doctor can reduce and possibly eliminate the drug treatment. If you get to a plateau, the dosage will be maintained at that point. Remember, even if you fall short of total drug-free treatment, you have still won if you have reduced drug dosage or simply gotten yourself in better physical and mental shape.

The major benefits you stand to gain include a reduction of drug side effects, lowering of some atherosclerotic risk factors, decreasing the workload imposed on the heart, and the indirect benefit of feeling better about yourself.

Will Step Zero work? There is no formula for predicting success, and many of the factors will be determined by the severity of your hypertension and end-organ damage, but if you can answer yes to the following questions, you are a good candidate:

- Are you interested in your health, and able to take direction?
- Will you be able to follow some relatively complex plans for diet and exercise?
- Do you have a strong motivation to take control of the situation?
- Are you able to exercise? Are you free of conditions that make walking painful?
- Are other factors under your control? For example, will it be reasonably convenient for you to follow a low-salt, low-calorie diet? Will other family members help you do it?

Another element to consider is the adaptability of your doctor to the program. While most if not all physicians will enthusiastically endorse diet, exercise, and stress control, working with a patient on a day-to-day basis is another story.

Remember, it is easier for a doctor to write a prescription for pills than it is for him or her to monitor your self-improvement efforts. It is also easier for *you* to simply swallow pills instead of dieting, running, and meditating. But even the most busy doctor-patient team will admit that the benefits can be worth the effort.

Case Histories

Not all cases are so cleanly solved as the following three, but they do illustrate what happens when Step Zero therapy works as it should.

CASE HISTORY 1

Mark is a forty-eight-year-old long-distance truck driver. He lived on a very poor, high-salt diet. In fact, his consumption of salt was about four times normal, primarily because he ate a great deal of highly salted soup. He would typically fill his thermos with soup before long drives, and would sip from the jug as he drove.

Mark was first seen in the office last summer because of a blood pressure check during a company physical; he was referred to this office by the company physician. Our physical showed a BP of 148/94.

The exam showed Mark to be thin and certainly not an overstressed individual. But on questioning, he revealed his salt intake. In addition to having salty soup, he typically ate a great deal of salted peanuts and pickles.

By simple elimination of those salty foods from his diet, Mark was able to lower his blood pressure within one month to 138/86.

He was surprised to realize how much salt he was taking in and how much that salt affected his blood pressure. Being an intelligent patient, he was able to significantly alter his salt intake, and at this point needs no further therapy.

CASE HISTORY 2

Jack is thirty-two years old, an executive, and was once an all-star college football player. During his playing days he weighed about 200 pounds and was trim and muscular.

However, he graduated to a desk job, and to compound matters he was recently married to a woman studying to be a chef. Last year his weight increased from 200 to 252 pounds.

Jack was referred to the office because his blood pressure registered 144/96 during a check made prior to a blood donation.

It was clear that his weight gain was due entirely to excess caloric intake. Jack was placed on a 1,000-calorie-per-day diet, to which he responded well. The patient lost almost 50 pounds in four months; at the same time his BP was lowered to 134/84.

He remains on Step Zero therapy with particular attention paid to exercise and diet.

CASE HISTORY 3

Louise is thirty-two years old, recently married, and was referred after a routine physical exam at her place of employment. Her BP was discovered to be 152/90.

The physical exam showed no nutritional or obesity problem. However, multiple bruises were observed on various parts of her body.

Under questioning, she admitted that her new husband was an alcoholic and beat her frequently. She was afraid to tell her family.

Louise was referred to a social service agency and has since left her husband. Within three weeks of leaving her husband, her blood pressure dropped to 120/80.

Again, things do not always work out so neatly. But these people—and they *are* real people—were able to work out their problems and uncover the aggravating factors of their hypertension. Perhaps you can too.

The Key to a Successful Step Zero Program

While we are reluctant to pass along any simple formulas—hypertension is a vastly complex problem, as you certainly are aware—one factor does predominate. In order to control your hypertension through drug-free therapy, you must *sincerely desire to improve your health.*

Desire is essential because the road ahead is not particularly easy. Diet and exercise take a great deal of motivation. Modifying any sort of behavior takes practice and dedication.

Things will be a little easier if you get help along the way. Try to involve your family and friends. Keep a record of your progress. One of the best tools for motivation is a graph showing weight declining and blood pressure dropping.

Basic Principles and Encouraging Words

To spur you along, let's discuss a final benefit of the programs outlined in the next three chapters. Just as various physical maladies interact to aggravate and magnify their individual consequences, so do health-producing regimens. Proper diet, physical conditioning, and stress reduction are synergistic—they interact and have an additive effect.

Exercise, for example, will help reduce stress. Rather than keeping all your frustrations in, it is much better to blow off some steam jogging or swimming. It is also thought that a program of vigorous exercise will reduce cholesterol and other fat levels in the blood.

Stress reduction not only reduces BP; it also lowers the heart rate. The best evidence indicates that a rapid heart rate puts you at much greater risk for coronary artery disease.

Diet works interactively with physical and psychological factors, too. The interaction of diet, exercise, and stress reduction will do more than improve a person's physique: It generally makes that person feel better about him- or herself. You *feel* better. Often, you will gain self-confidence and be able to convert stressful situations into nonstress situations. Possibly, your new approach will make you more energetic and productive in your personal and professional life.

Chapters 5, 6, and 7 will deal with diet, exercise, and stress reduction, respectively. Those chapters will expand on the general information presented in this chapter, and we will spell out some proven strategies. Before moving on, here are some of the questions often posed about the general subject of drug-free antihypertensive therapy:

Q: I would really like to take off some weight fast. Will the diet plans in the next chapter help?

A: Yes, but the emphasis will be on permanent weight control rather than crash dieting. There is a good reason for this: It appears that atherosclerosis is aggravated by weight gain but not alleviated to the same degree by weight loss. This means that up-and-down weight cycles can be harmful.

Q: Does hypertension itself preclude any particular types of exercise?

A: If the medications you are taking make you subject to postural hypotension (a drastic drop in blood pressure when you get to your feet quickly), certain activities, especially those involving up-and-down motion, will have to be modified.

Q: I encounter stressful situations at various times during the day, but I generally get it out of my system and get back to normal. So I do not think my high blood pressure is a long-term thing. Can isolated episodes of stress hurt me?

A: Yes. The best and most recent evidence indicates that the occasional rapid rise of blood pressure is damaging, too. The subject is covered in greater detail in the entry on labile hypertension in Chapter 8.

[5]
Lowering
Blood Pressure
through Diet

While scientists and researchers are less than clear on many of the factors influencing hypertension in particular and longevity in general, there is one risk factor that we *know* is critical to both: controlling body weight.

The vast preponderance of evidence shows that BP rises when body weight is up, and falls when body weight is down. In one study, each 1 percent increase in body weight was accompanied by a 1 percent increase in blood pressure.

Obesity in the United States is a major problem, not only in the treatment of hypertension but in the treatment of all cardiovascular problems. It is estimated that one third of men over the age of thirty and one fifth of women over that age are 30 percent or more over ideal body weight. Anywhere from 20 to 30 percent over ideal body weight is considered by most physicians to constitute overweight.

We will get to that so-called ideal weight in a minute, but first let's talk about body fat and hypertension. To begin with, the effect is more pronounced in the systolic reading; that is, the systolic reading is more directly increased by body weight than is the diastolic reading. For women, there is generally a closer relationship between body weight and hypertension than for men, especially in cases where a woman is less than sixty years of age and has a family history of hypertension.

Incidentally, be aware that blood pressure readings on obese patients can be inaccurate if the doctor (or patient doing blood pressure self-monitoring) uses too small a cuff. Obese patients with very large arms need a cuff commonly used to take BP on the thigh.

The precise reason why increased body fat elevates blood pressure—and why decreased fat lowers pressure—is not totally understood. It is currently thought that weight loss is related to a decrease in the amount of blood the heart must pump and a decrease in the resistance offered to blood flow throughout the body. These two factors, the heart working less hard and less resistance in the system, apparently combine to lower the blood pressure.

As far as the effect of weight itself, here are some facts that may—and *should*—scare you:

- If you are a middle-aged man who is 30 percent overweight you have *four times* the risk, as compared to a man of normal body weight, of having coronary artery disease and *seven times* the risk of having a stroke.
- To make things worse, there is a direct relationship between obesity and elevated cholesterol. When an obese individual finally eats himself onto the autospy table, the pathologist will typically find deposits clogging the coronary vessels. (More details on cholesterol are in a following section of this chapter.)
- The pathologist will also find an enlarged heart and evidence of high blood pressure in the circulatory system. Not a pretty sight—but a sight we have seen with distressing regularity.

The hypertensive, of course, has to be concerned with diet in areas other than simple weight loss. Salt is traditionally reduced in the diet for a hypertensive, although it is important to point out that many cases of hypertension will not respond much if at all to salt reduction. This, of course, relates to the root cause of the hypertension. Someone with the type of volume-related hypertension described in earlier chapters may respond quite sharply to salt reduction. A patient whose problem stems from an oversupply of renin might not lower his blood pressure reading at all, even with practically all salt eliminated from the diet.

Still, sensible salt reduction is always worthwhile, as is control of cholesterol and triglycerides, a group of fatty substances that are found in the blood. Cholesterol and triglycerides are found in foods, and to an extent their presence in the blood is controlled by how much of them we eat. However, our liver produces these substances, too. An out-of-whack metabolism can overload your body with cholesterol and/or triglycerides even if your consumption is next to nil.

Some research indicates that potassium chloride and potassium—which are found in a variety of foods—have a controlling effect on hypertension.

A big problem faced by hypertensives is the apparent complexity of their recommended diet(s), and the fact that many health professionals have neither the time nor the inclination to explain *what* is happening because of food intake, and *why* it happens. Too often, the patient gets a recommendation to "cut down on the cholesterol" when he or she does not have any idea of what cholesterol is or where it is found. In some cases, the recommendation is to "watch the salt," but no explanation is given concerning sources of hidden salt. And if losing weight were really that simple, we would all look like greyhounds; thinness has become a national obsession.

This chapter will demystify diets and dieting. We will start with the simple foundation of a hypertensive's diet—salt reduction, an action that can produce immediate benefits—and move on to weight loss, a longer-term goal but probably the most important in terms of your overall health. Once we have hammered together the framework of salt reduction and weight control, the next item will be an explanation of blood fat (including cholesterol) levels—what they mean and how they are monitored. Also, we will take a look at some of the newest theories concerning foods that appear to have an antihypertensive effect.

Sodium Reduction

So, what's the story on salt? Is it really the root of hypertension, or is that a disproven belief? The answers are: maybe, and maybe.

To understand the salt story, let's define a few basic terms and processes. The terms "salt" and "sodium" are frequently used interchangeably, but they have different meanings. Salt, in common usage, means *sodium chloride*, a naturally occurring white crystal that has roughly 40 percent sodium and 60 percent chloride. Using basic math, then, if you are eating five grams of salt per day in your food you are really taking in two grams of sodium. (A gram is roughly a third of an ounce, about the weight of a paper clip.)

Before you condemn sodium altogether, bear in mind that you need it to live. Sodium is responsible for maintaining the proper blood volume, keeping various fluid levels in the body at appropriate levels, and making cell membranes strong and resilient. Sodium also plays a role in transmitting nerve impulses, and aids in the contraction of muscle tissue, including the heart.

The body has an intricate system for maintaining the proper level of sodium in the blood. Too little sodium coming in? The body makes you crave salty foods. Without *any* sodium, you would eventually go into shock and die (although such a severe sodium shortage would be extremely difficult to achieve with the types of food generally offered for sale these days).

Too much sodium in the system? No problem! The body asks you to dilute the sodium so it can be excreted. (In other words, salty food makes you thirsty, which is no surprise to tavern owners who serve salted peanuts at the bar.) But those of us with volume-dependent hypertension cannot excrete sodium so easily. Sodium stays in our system and keeps the fluid volume high. Hypertension results. To explain it another way, when we eat too much sodium, the kidney causes the body to retain fluid, which soaks the tissues and sometimes produces puffy swelling, and also raises the amount of fluid in the vascular system. In people whose fluid-balance systems are working correctly, the fluid retention is not extreme, and the fluid—along with the extra sodium—is soon excreted. But certain hypertensives have highly reactive fluid levels and can not get that sodium or extra fluid out of their systems efficiently.

In the United States we tend to eat a lot of sodium. Most nutritionists feel that an average adult needs between 1 and 3 grams of sodium in the diet per day. But we customarily eat between 5 and 15 grams a day, according to some estimates.

There is a body of thought that holds excess sodium responsible for most cases of hypertension. After all, if you feed lab animals huge amounts of salt, their blood pressure will rise. Secondly, statistical studies of populations with high dietary sodium intake typically show marked BP elevations in the populations.

But not everyone is a sodium reactor. Some people can ingest huge amounts of sodium and keep a stable pressure. On the other hand, some hypertensives can eliminate a great deal of sodium from the diet and not bring about a reduced reading. So while salt reduction does not appear to be the high-blood-pressure panacea it was once thought to be, it still is a major part of most people's antihypertension program.

It certainly will be mandatory for a sodium reactor, the person who retains fluid because he or she cannot excrete sodium properly. This is a factor your doctor will take into account during a physical exam. If your ankles and wrists are swollen, for example, that is a pretty good indication that you are a sodium reactor. A puffy face (though not necessarily a fat face—sodium reactors can be thin) is another telltale. A sodium-reactive person typically responds well to diuretics, which help flush the sodium *and* the excess fluid out of the system.

The big question, then, is how much sodium should be eliminated from the diet? And how do you do it? In general, you probably will want to strive for that 1 to 3 grams of sodium per day. And the most effective way to do this is to *eliminate discretionary use of salt and find the hidden salt* in your diet.

First, realize that you cannot walk around with a pocket calculator and add up every last milligram of sodium you put in your mouth. A rigid approach like this is doomed to fail; a biochemist probably could not do it. Instead, you must become aware of the approximate salt levels of various foods and adjust your eating habits accordingly. Start by getting an idea of where that sodium is—and in what amounts. Table 1 lists common foods according to their sodium, potassium, and caloric content. All those values will eventually prove useful as we plan an antihypertensive diet, and we will refer back to this table several times.

Note that the values for sodium and potassium are expressed in milligrams (mg)—thousandths of a gram. One thousand milligrams equals one gram. As an example, one cup of corned beef hash is listed as containing 1,188 mg of sodium, or 1.188 grams. If your goal is to keep sodium intake between 1 and 3 grams, canned corned beef hash is a good thing to avoid, since one cup will use up a third of your maximum daily allowance.

Be aware that foods do not have to *taste* salty to have high sodium levels. For example, a regular order of fast-food-restaurant french fries, while they taste salty, can have four times *less* sodium than the same restaurant's serving of cherry pie. This surprising fact stems from the use of salt (sodium chloride) as part of food processing, along with substances such as sodium saccharin, sodium nitrite, sodium ascorbate, sodium benzoate, monosodium glutamate, and all those other appe-

Table 1. Sodium, Potassium, and Caloric Content of Foods (All figures are approximate and may vary depending on brand name, manufacturer, food processor, or actual size of item.)

BREADS, ROLLS, ETC.	Amount	Mg Sodium	Mg Potassium	Calories
White	1 slice	142	29	76
Rye	1 slice	139	36	61
Whole wheat	1 slice	132	68	61
Biscuit	1 (2" diameter)	185	18	104
Cornbread	2½" square	263	61	178
Frankfurter roll	both halves	202	38	119
Hamburger roll	both halves	202	38	119
Pancake	1 (6" diameter)	412	112	164
Waffle	1 (7" diameter)	515	146	206
Graham crackers	2 (2½" squares)	95	55	55
Brown rice	1 cup (cooked with salt)	550	137	232
White rice	1 cup (cooked with salt)	767	57	223
Bran flakes	1 cup	207	137	106
Corn flakes	1 cup	251	30	97
Oatmeal	1 cup (cooked)	523	146	132
Puffed rice	1 cup	148	33	140
Wheat flakes	1 cup	310	81	106
Flour, wheat	1 cup (all purpose)	130	0	499
Egg noodles	1 cup	3	70	200
Macaroni	1 cup	1	103	192
Spaghetti	1 cup	1	103	192

FRUITS	Amount	Mg Sodium	Mg Potassium	Calories
Apple	1 (2½" diameter)	1	116	61
Apricots, fresh	3 medium	1	301	55
Apricots, dried	5 large halves	6	235	62
Banana	1 medium	1	440	101
Blackberries	1 cup	1	245	84
Cantaloupe	½ (5" diameter)	33	682	82
Cherries, sweet	10	1	129	47
Dates	10	1	518	219
Fig	1 large	1	126	52
Grapefruit	½ small	1	132	40
Grapes	1 cup	3	160	70
Honeydew	½ (6½" diameter)	90	1,881	247
Orange	1 medium	1	290	66
Peach	1 (2¾" diameter	2	308	58
Pear	1 (2½" diameter)	3	213	100
Pineapple	1 cup	2	226	81
Plum	1 (1" diameter)	Trace	30	7
Prunes, dried	10 medium	5	448	164
Raisins	1 tablespoon	2	69	26
Raspberries, black	1 cup	1	267	98
Strawberries	1 cup	1	244	55
Tangerine	1 (2⅜" diameter)	2	108	39
Watermelon	1 cup	2	160	42

Table 1, *continued*

DAIRY PRODUCTS	Amount	Mg Sodium	Mg Potassium	Calories
American cheese	1 slice	322	23	105
Blue cheese dressing	1 tablespoon	164	6	76
Cheddar cheese	1 slice	147	17	84
Cottage cheese, low-fat	1 cup	580	144	172
Cream cheese	1 cup	580	172	868
Parmesan cheese	1 oz	208	42	111
Swiss cheese	1 oz	201	29	105
Butter (salted)	1 stick	1,119	26	812
Butter (unsalted)	1 stick	<1	<1	812
Buttermilk	1 cup	319	343	88
Skim milk	1 cup	127	355	88
Whole milk	1 cup	122	351	159
Evaporated milk	1 cup	297	764	345
Heavy cream	1 tablespoon	5	13	53
Ice cream (no salt)	1 cup	84	241	257
Hot chocolate	1 cup	120	370	238
Hot cocoa	1 cup	128	363	243
Egg yolk	1 medium	8	15	52
Egg white	1 medium	42	40	15
Egg, fried	1 medium	135	56	86
Egg, boiled	1 medium	54	57	72
Egg, scrambled	1 medium	144	82	97
Yogurt, plain	1 cup	115	323	152

MEAT AND POULTRY	Amount	Mg Sodium	Mg Potassium	Calories
BEEF				
Corned beef hash	1 cup, canned	1,188	440	398
Frankfurter	1 medium	627	125	176
Heart	1 oz	29	66	53
Hamburger	2.9 oz, lean	49	221	235
Kidney	1 cup	354	454	353
Liver, beef	3 oz	156	323	195
Rib roast	10¾ oz	149	680	1,342
Flank steak	3 oz	45	207	167
Porterhouse steak	10.6 oz	145	664	1,400
Sirloin steak	10.9 oz	173	793	1,192
T-Bone steak	10.4 oz	141	644	1,395
LAMB				
Chop	1 medium	51	234	341
Roast	3 oz	60	273	158
PORK				
Bacon	1 slice	123	29	72
Chops, shoulder cut	3 oz	47	214	300
Ham, baked	3 oz	770	241	159
Roast	3 oz	698	218	281
Spareribs	6.3 oz	65	299	792
VEAL				
Cutlets	3 oz	56	258	184
Calves' liver	3 oz	100	385	222
Loin cut	9.5 oz	174	795	629
Roast	3 oz	57	259	229
Sweetbreads	3 oz	*	*	143

*Adequate data not available.

Table 1, *continued*

MEAT AND POULTRY, continued	Amount	Mg Sodium	Mg Potassium	Calories
CHICKEN				
A La King	1 cup	760	404	468
Broiled	7.1 oz	133	551	273
Liver, chopped	1 cup	85	211	231
Light meat	1 piece, 2½" x 1⅞" x ¼"	16	103	42
Dark meat	1 piece, 1⅞" x 1" x ¼"	9	32	18
TURKEY				
White meat	2 pieces 4" x 2" x ¼"	70	349	150
Dark meat	2 pieces 2½" x 1⅝" x ½"	42	169	87

FRESH VEGETABLES	Amount	Mg Sodium	Mg Potassium	Calories
Asparagus	1 cup	3	375	35
Beans, lima	1 cup	3	1,008	191
Beets	1 cup	81	452	58
Broccoli	1 lb	68	1,733	145
Carrot	1 medium	34	246	30
Celery	1 stalk	50	136	7
Corn, sweet	1 ear (no butter or salt)	Trace	151	70
Cucumber	1 large, 8¼" long	18	481	45
Eggplant	1 cup, cooked	2	300	38
Lettuce, iceberg	1 head (6" diameter)	48	943	70
Onion	1 cup, chopped	17	267	65
Peas	1 cup	3	458	122
Potato, baked	1 medium	6	782	145
Potato, boiled	1 medium	4	556	104
Radishes	10 large	15	261	14
Spinach	1 cup	39	259	14
Sweet potato	1 medium, boiled	15	367	172
Tomato	1 medium	4	300	27
Watercress	1 cup	18	99	7

FRESH FISH AND SEAFOOD	Amount	Mg Sodium	Mg Potassium	Calories
Bass, striped	3 oz	*	*	168
Clams, cherrystone	4 clams	144	218	56
Cod	3 oz	93	345	144
Crab	1 cup	*	*	144
Flounder	3 oz	201	498	171
Haddock	3 oz	150	297	141
Halibut	3 oz	114	447	144
Lobster	1 cup	305	261	138
Mackerel	3 oz	*	*	201
Oysters	3 small	21	34	19
Salmon	3 oz	99	378	156
Shrimp	3 oz	159	195	192

*Adequate data not available.

98

Table 1, *continued*

CANNED VEGETABLES*	Amount	Mg Sodium	Mg Potassium	Calories
Asparagus	14½ oz can	970	682	74
Beans, green	8 oz can	536	216	41
Beans, lima	8½ oz can	1,070	1,007	322
Beets	8 oz can	535	379	77
Carrots	8 oz can	535	272	64
Corn, creamed	8¾ oz can	585	241	203
Peas	8½ oz can	569	231	159
Spinach	7¾ oz can	519	550	42
Tomatoes	16 oz can	590	984	95

*Some specially marked canned goods are processed without added salt and may be suitable for low-salt diets. Check the labels.

SWEETS	Amount	Mg Sodium	Mg Potassium	Calories
Angel food cake	½12 cake	170	53	161
Brownie	1¾" x 1¾" x ⅞"	50	38	97
Chocolate, bittersweet	1 oz	1	174	135
Chocolate cupcake	1 (2½" diameter)	74	35	92
Chocolate chip cookies	10 (2¼" diameter)	421	141	495
Chocolate syrup	1 oz	20	106	92
Gelatin, sweet	3 oz	270	*	315
Honey	1 tablespoon	1	11	64
Jelly	1 tablespoon	3	14	49
Sherbet, orange	1 cup	19	42	259
Sponge cake	½12 cake	110	57	196
Sugar, brown	1 cup	44	499	541
Sugar, granulated	1 cup	2	6	770
Sugar, powdered	1 cup	1	4	462

*Adequate data not available.

BEVERAGES	Amount	Mg Sodium	Mg Potassium	Calories
Coffee, instant	1 teaspoon	1	29	1
Coffee, regular	1 cup	2	65	2
Beer	8 oz	17	60	101
Gin, Rye, Rum, Scotch, Vodka	1 oz 80 proof	Trace	1	65
	1 oz 86 proof	Trace	1	70
	1 oz 90 proof	Trace	1	74
	1 oz 94 proof	Trace	1	77
	1 oz 100 proof	Trace	1	83
Sherry	2 oz	2	44	81

FRUIT JUICES (Canned or bottled)	Amount	Mg Sodium	Mg Potassium	Calories
Apple	1 cup	2	250	117
Apricot nectar	1 cup	Trace	379	143
Cranberry	1 cup	3	25	164
Grape	1 cup	5	293	167
Grapefruit (unsweetened)	1 cup	2	400	101
Lemon	1 tablespoon	Trace	43	7
Orange (fresh)	1 cup	2	496	112
Pineapple (unsweetened)	1 cup	3	373	138
Prune	1 cup	5	602	197
Tomato	1 cup	486	552	46

HIGH SODIUM FOODS

FLAVORS, BLENDS, AND SEASONINGS

Bouillon cubes	Gelatin, flavored	Onion salt
Candies	Horseradish with salt	Pickles
Catsup	Mayonnaise	Pudding mixes
Celery salt	Meat extracts	Relish
Celery flakes	Meat sauces	Rennet tablets
Chili sauce	Meat tenderizers	Salt
French dressing	Molasses	Salted nuts
Garlic salt	Mustard	Salt or sugar substitutes
	Olives	Soy sauce
		Worchestershire sauce

BEVERAGES

All canned soups*	Chocolate milk	Milk shakes
Cocoa instant mixes	Malted milk	Salted buttermilk

MEATS

All canned meats, soups, and stews*	Frankfurters	Salted meat
Bacon	Ham	Salt pork
Bologna	Kidneys	Sausage
Brains	Liverwurst	Smoked meat
Chipped beef	Pickled meat	Spiced meat
Corned beef	Salami	

MISCELLANEOUS

All canned fish*	Salted cheeses
All canned vegetables*	Salted ice cream and sherbet
All salted fish	Salted butter
All shellfish	Salted buttermilk
All smoked fish	Salted popcorn, potato chips, and pretzels
Anchovies	
Caviar	

*Some specially marked canned goods are processed without added salt and may be suitable for low-salt diets. Check the labels.

FOOD ADDITIVES HIGH IN SODIUM

Baking powder	Sodium bicarbonate
Brine	Sodium benzoate
Di-sodium phosphate	Sodium chloride (salt)
Monosodium glutamate	Sodium hydroxide
Sodium (Na)	Sodium propionate
Sodium alginate	Sodium sulfite

Source: <u>Nutritive Value of American Foods in Common Units.</u> Agricultural Handbook No. 456. Agricultural Research Service, 1975.

Reprinted from "The Hypertensives' Guide for a Balanced Diet," courtesy of Ayerst Laboratories.

tizing ingredients you see listed on the labels of packaged foods. These chemicals are added to enhance flavor, lengthen shelf life, and cut costs.

If you do not take hidden sodium into account, your sodium-reduction diet will most likely fail.

You will note from Table 1 that heavily processed and canned foods are typically high in sodium. That is generally a good guide even if you cannot locate a sodium listing on the label.

Fast food is typically heavy in sodium. A large hamburger with cheese can easily top 1 gram of sodium. TV dinners are high, too, often containing a gram of sodium or more.

Sodium hides in other places. A dose of Alka Seltzer has 532 mg of sodium. The water you drink may contain a high amount of sodium. In New York State, for example, sodium content of water can legally be as high as 220 mg per liter of water.

So, what to do? Sodium seems to lurk everywhere and would appear to be inextricable from the typical American diet. There is, unfortunately, a milligram of truth in that statement. It would be very difficult to keep a running track of all sodium intake, and next to impossible to keep that sodium low if you subsist on canned foods, TV dinners, and fast-food hamburgers. But you *can* take a simple, common-sense approach to the problem and cut back on sodium as much as you reasonably can.

Here is what you can do:

1. Learn which foods are high in sodium. Read labels on foods and refer to the sodium chart in Table 1. Some foods have their sodium content listed on the can or the box; with others you will have to rely on the chart. In any case, you know that *canned, highly processed, or fast foods* are generally not a good bet; avoid them. (Canned fruits and fruit juices, though, are OK.) Specifically avoid the items listed as "High Sodium Foods" in Table 1.
2. Eliminate salt from the table. One teaspoon of table salt contains about two grams of sodium. Use commercially available salt substitutes, such as potassium chloride (no sodium, the best option) or "low-salt" (reduced-sodium chloride).

3. Eliminate salt from your cooking. If you think food tastes too bland when cooked without salt, try using herbs and spices. Buy individual, unsalted spices, not the prepared, salted mixtures. If calories are not restricted, you may use jam, jelly, honey, unsalted butter, and low-sodium salad dressing. Fresh fruit may also be used to enhance the flavor of your meals. Here are some flavoring suggestions for a wide variety of foods:

MEAT, FISH, AND EGGS

BEEF—allspice, basil, bay leaf, cardamon, chives, curry, garlic, grape or currant jelly, lemon juice, mace, marjoram, mushrooms, dry mustard, nutmeg, onion, oregano, paprika, parsley, pepper, green peppers, sage, savory, tarragon, thyme, turmeric, vinegar or wine for marinating.

PORK—apples, applesauce, basil, cardamon, cloves, curry, cranberries, dill, fruit juices, garlic, mace, marjoram, dry mustard, oregano, onion, parsley, pepper, pineapple, rosemary, sage, thyme, turmeric

LAMB—basil, curry, dill, garlic, mace, marjoram, mint, onion, oregano, parsley, pepper, pineapple rings, rosemary, thyme, turmeric

VEAL—apricots, basil, bay leaf, current jelly, curry, dill, garlic, ginger, mace, marjoram, oregano, paprika, parsley, peaches, pepper, rosemary, sage, savory, tarragon, thyme, turmeric

CHICKEN OR TURKEY—allspice, basil, bay leaf, cardamon, cranberry sauce, cumin, curry, garlic, mace, marjoram, mushrooms, dry mustard, paprika, parsley, pepper, pineapple sauce, rosemary, sage, savory, tarragon, thyme, turmeric

FISH—bay leaf, chives, coriander, curry, dill, garlic, lemon juice, mace, marjoram, mushrooms, dry mustard, onion, oregano, paprika, parsley, pepper, green peppers, sage, savory, tarragon, thyme, turmeric

EGGS—basil, chili powder, chives, cumin, curry, mace, marjoram, mushrooms, dry mustard, jelly or pineapple omelet, onion, paprika, parsley, pepper, green peppers, rosemary, savory, tarragon, thyme.

VEGETABLES

ASPARAGUS—caraway seed, lemon juice, dry mustard, unsalted chopped nuts, nutmeg, sesame seeds.

BROCCOLI—lemon juice, oregano, tarragon.

CABBAGE—basil, unsalted butter with lemon and sugar, caraway seed, cinnamon, dill, mace, dry mustard, nutmeg, savory, tarragon.

CARROTS—butter, glazed with unsalted butter and sugar, chili powder, cinnamon, ginger, mace, marjoram, mint, nutmeg, parsley, poppy seed, thyme.

CAULIFLOWER—caraway seeds, curry, dill, mace, nutmeg, rosemary, savory, tarragon.

CORN—chili powder, chives, curry, parsley, green peppers, pimento, tomatoes.

GREEN BEANS—slivered almonds, basil, bay leaves, dill, cinnamon, lemon juice, mace, marjoram, nutmeg, onion, oregano, rosemary, sesame.

PEAS—chili powder, cinnamon, dill, mace, marjoram, mint, mushrooms, dry mustard, onion, oregano, parsley, green peppers, poppy seed, savory, thyme.

POTATOES—unsalted butter, caraway seed, chives, dill, mace, mint, oregano, onion, parsley, green peppers, poppy seed, thyme.

SQUASH—basil, ginger, mace, marjoram, onion, oregano.

SWEET POTATO—allspice, cardamon, ginger, brown sugar, candied or glazed with cinnamon or nutmeg, escalloped with apples, sugar, or orange slices.

TOMATOES—basil, chives, dill, marjoram, onion, oregano, parsley, sage, sugar, tarragon, thyme.

If you must add salt while cooking or to table food, taste the food first to see if it really needs it. Do not add salt as a habit.

4. Weight the odds in your favor by *adding* foods low in sodium. Fresh or frozen vegetables, fresh fish, and fresh, frozen, or canned fruits and juices are typically good choices.

5. Keep on the alert for hidden sodium. In particular, read the labels of antacids for sodium content. Do not be reluctant to ask your

doctor about sodium content of medications. Scrutinize other nonfood items, such as carbonated beverages.

6. In restaurants, avoid foods with sauces. Ask the waiter to have your food prepared without added salt.

Gauging your sodium intake will come with practice. Once you are conversant with sodium levels, keep an approximate total of sodium intake by writing down *everything* you eat for one day and determining, to the best of your ability, the sodium level. If it is still too high, back off a bit.

Some people are more successful with a stringent, predetermined diet plan. If you do not think you can lower sodium on your own, a low-sodium diet is provided in Appendix A. You may elect to try this diet even if you eventually plan to make up your own low-sodium plan, since it will give you an idea of the strategy of low sodium eating.

In any event, make your goal *reasonable sodium reduction over the long term.*

A superrestrictive plan may be unrealistic and counterproductive simply because you probably would not stick to it and you would return to your old eating habits. Unless your doctor tells you that immediate and drastic sodium reduction is critical, experiment and learn the best routine for *you*. And if you slip off the plan, get back on it. One case of backsliding will not ruin everything. Just cut back a little more closely on sodium in the next day's intake and then level off.

You have noticed that Table 1 also contains a listing of potassium. Potassium is particularly important to hypertensives for two reasons:

1. It is a substance needed by the body but often flushed out by diuretics.
2. A substance called potassium chloride, which is typically found with potassium, may, according to some recent evidence, have a protective effect against hypertension.

The subject of potassium washout and the need for supplementation will be addressed in Chapter 8. However, be aware at this point that many people can keep adequate potassium in their systems simply by eating foods high in that metallic element.

You can accomplish two goals at once by adding foods to your diet that are low in sodium and high in potassium. Eating generous amounts of these foods can help avoid a potassium deficiency. Some recommendations from the American Heart Association:

Foods High in Potassium, Low in Sodium
(Foods listed in CAPITAL LETTERS are especially helpful)

FRUITS

Apple, apricot, AVOCADO, BANANA, CANTALOUPE, date, grapefruit, HONEYDEW MELON, NECTARINE, prune, RAISIN, watermelon, apple juice, GRAPEFRUIT JUICE, prune juice, orange juice

VEGETABLES

Asparagus, beans—white or green, broccoli, brussel sprouts, cabbage (cooked), cauliflower (cooked), corn-on-the-cob, eggplant (cooked), lima beans (fresh and cooked), peas—green (fresh and cooked), peppers, POTATOES (BAKED or BOILED), radishes, squash—summer and winter (cooked).

Unfortunately, some foods that are relatively high in potassium are also high in sodium. *Limit* or *avoid* these: canned or bottled tomato juice, raw clams, sardines, frozen lima beans, frozen peas, canned spinach, canned carrots.

While life on a low-sodium diet involves some thought and effort, it is really not as complex as it might, at first, seem. Granted, if you must immediately drop to negligible amounts of sodium and calculate every milligram that passes your palate, the going will be rough for a while. Every new method of doing something takes time to learn.

However, you can learn to live with much less salt and—believe it or not—you will like the taste of your food better once you get out of the habit of eating highly processed foods and dumping salt on everything. You will find, for example, that plain baked potatoes are delicious. This is something you might not be aware of because in this culture we typically use the poor potato as nothing more than a vehicle for butter, salt, and sour cream.

So take a few days to ease yourself into a low-sodium diet. Learn all you can about low-sodium foods, and resolve to eat as much food as possible in a state where it has undergone the *minimum amount of processing*.

And use that salt shaker as a paperweight.

Weight Control

It is easy to talk about weight loss. For that matter, it is easy to *write* about weight loss. The hard part is actually losing the weight.

There are no "miracle" weight loss programs, and the fact that a desperate person may over a lifetime clutch at dozens—maybe hundreds—of purported "easy" methods is a sad commentary on our gullibility and short memories.

To risk sounding as though we are advocating our own miracle diet, we would like to propose some theories about why people do not lose weight when they want to and/or need to. Essentially, most folks who fail repeatedly on diets do not understand that losing weight and keeping that weight off involves:

1. Reduction in calories
2. Exercise
3. Behavioral modification

Point number 3 is, in the long run, the most important. Without modifying the way we eat and the way we view food, we really cannot undertake a successful diet program. Eating is a habit as well as a method of life-support. People who are unable to control their weight have developed some bad eating habits; they must learn to alter how fast they eat, what type of foods they eat, and their eating lifestyle (at home vs. on the run, set mealtimes vs. snacking, etc.).

They must also take a positive attitude toward weight control, convincing themselves that when they lose weight they will feel better, look better, and live longer. And if you are not convinced that weight loss will help you live longer, consider that many "ideal" weight tables are published by life insurance companies (Table 2).

One of the major roadblocks encountered by frustrated dieters is that they go about weight loss in a backward fashion: They try to reduce food intake without establishing a baseline. In other words, they do not know how much food they need to take in to maintain present weight and how much they need to take away to lose weight.

Here is a plan that may seem hopelessly vague by the standards of the current popular media. We can not—and would not—give you a

Table 2. Height and Weight

Weights at ages 25–59 based on lowest mortality. Weight in pounds according to frame (in indoor clothing weighing 5 lbs. for men and 3 lbs. for women; shoes with 1″ heels).

MEN · **WOMEN**

Height Feet Inches	Small Frame	Medium Frame	Large Frame	Height Feet Inches	Small Frame	Medium Frame	Large Frame
5 2	128-134	131-141	138-150	4 10	102-111	109-121	118-131
5 3	130-136	133-143	140-153	4 11	103-113	111-123	120-134
5 4	132-138	135-145	142-156	5 0	104-115	113-126	122-137
5 5	134-140	137-148	144-160	5 1	106-118	115-129	125-140
5 6	136-142	139-151	146-164	5 2	108-121	118-132	128-143
5 7	138-145	142-154	149-168	5 3	111-124	121-135	131-147
5 8	140-148	145-157	152-172	5 4	114-127	124-138	134-151
5 9	142-151	148-160	155-176	5 5	117-130	127-141	137-155
5 10	144-154	151-163	158-180	5 6	120-133	130-144	140-159
5 11	146-157	154-166	161-184	5 7	123-136	133-147	143-163
6 0	149-160	157-170	164-188	5 8	126-139	136-150	146-167
6 1	152-164	160-174	168-192	5 9	129-142	139-153	149-170
6 2	155-168	164-178	172-197	5 10	132-145	142-156	152-173
6 3	158-172	167-182	176-202	5 11	135-148	145-159	155-176
6 4	162-176	171-187	181-207	6 0	138-151	148-162	158-179

Reprinted, courtesy of Metropolitan Life Insurance Company, from "1983 Metropolitan Height and Weight Tables." Source of basic data: *1979 Build Study,* Society of Actuaries and Association of Life Insurance Medical Directors of America, 1980.

regimen that guarantees that you will lose two pounds a day by drinking an herbal tea or taking a fruit extract pill. Instead, we want you to design *your own* diet plan.

Why a plan of your own making? Because you are going to have to stick within the framework of your diet for the rest of your life. You may *lose* weight on a diet utilizing foods you detest, but once that diet is over, you will be a sure bet to return to your old eating habits.

So instead of putting yourself back on the frustrating (and physically damaging) cycle of weight loss and weight regain, try this plan:

1. First, find out approximately how many calories you need to maintain your present weight. One simple way to figure out how many calories you need per day to maintain present weight is to take your weight and multiply it by 12 to 14 if you are a woman

or 14 to 16 if you are a man. The resulting figure will show how many calories you must eat per day to maintain that weight.

2. Now that you have an idea of what level maintains your weight, cut back. Use the figures in Table 1, or other calorie counters of your choice, to remove 500 or 1,000 calories a day from your diet. Since a pound of fat generally is put around your waistline by an excess calorie intake of 3,500 calories, a reduction of 500 calories a day for seven days equals a one-pound weight loss.

To put it in arithmetically:

$$(500 \text{ calories less per day}) \times (7 \text{ days})$$
$$= 3,500 \text{ calories less per week}$$

Since:

3,500 calories = one pound, cutting back 500 calories a day = a one pound per week weight loss.

So, by removing a few items a day—a couple of donuts, say—you can get those 500 calories out of your system and lose about a pound a week. Cutting back by 1,000 calories per day can translate to two pounds a week.

Do not go too low, because placing yourself in a state of semistarvation produces diminishing returns; your body thinks you have been shipwrecked without provisions and lowers its metabolism to cope with the extreme deprivation and conserve calories during the emergency.

For most of us, the lowest permissible calorie level should not go much below 1,500 calories a day, but small and inactive people may need a further reduction to promote steady weight loss.

A slow, steady loss is usually preferable to a fast loss, because the weight taken off slowly tends to stay off. One or two pounds a week is a good goal.

Incidentally, you can opt to eat the same number of calories and lose a pound per week by exercising it off, but it takes a lot of effort. To expend 500 calories per day, you must bicycle for one and one-half hours a day, or run for forty-five minutes per day, or play tennis for an hour per day or golf for two hours per day.

3. Keep some foods you like in your diet, but eliminate foods high in sodium and dense in calories. Gradually introduce some more healthful foods into your diet. For example, you may think salads are a good addition to a weight control plan, and you are right. But if you do not eat salads now, and do not particularly like them, do not force yourself into a rabbit-food regimen of salad, salad, and more salad. Add a salad to your dinner menu twice a week, and experiment with various salad recipes until you find one you like. Stick to this plan and you will probably end up liking salads more than frozen pizza. Fresh, unprocessed food is very pleasing to the palate once you become accustomed to it.

4. Work to balance your diet among the food groups. Food groups are usually broken down into fruits, vegetables, grains, dairy products, and meat-fish-poultry, although individual diet plans break down food groupings into various categories and subcategories.

   What you eventually want is a flexible diet plan that allows substitution from among various food groups. This takes away some of the monotony and balances your nutrient intake. Appendix B contains a sample reducing diet based on the substitution list theory. You may wish to try this diet if your physician recommends a very quick program of weight loss or if you do not have the desire to design your own plan.

5. Now comes the hard part. Stay on your diet and keep the weight off once you lose it. This can only be done by changing your eating habits. Here are some suggestions:

   - If you have trouble controlling snacking, change your schedule so that you are busy at the time you usually snack. You may not even notice the hunger pangs.
   - Control your hunger pangs by delaying gratification. If you feel hungry, wait for twenty minutes before snacking. If you continue to do this—make it a habit—your hunger pangs may simply fade away or at least be easier to ignore.
   - When eating, be sure that all you do is eat. If you are watching TV or reading during a meal, you will not really

enjoy the food. Make eating a time of enjoyment: Enjoy the taste of each bite and make eating a conscious act.

- Eat slowly. Double the amount of time it takes to eat. Set your fork down between bites.
- Reward yourself for being successful. Give yourself money, or time off, or best of all, new and smaller clothes.
- Try to identify what emotions trigger your desire to eat. Recognize the fact that you may eat a bag of cookies because you are lonely, or bored—not because you are particularly hungry. When you experience cravings, recognize that there may be a conditioned reflex at work and ask yourself, "Why do I really want these cookies?"
- Do not keep junk food handy and easily available.
- Eat in the same place and at the same time each day.
- Be active. While you cannot rely on exercise alone to burn off fat, it helps in more ways than one.

One final note on weight control for the hypertensive: Be sure to avoid over-the-counter appetite suppressants, since most elevate blood pressure.

Cholesterol and Triglycerides

While the primary cause of atherosclerosis is unknown, the presence of high levels of fatty substances (lipids) in the blood appears to be, along with hypertension, one of the major culprits.

Popular usage has given cholesterol and triglycerides the same type of connotation as "snake bite" and "tax audit." However, these substances are not necessarily poisonous or damaging. In fact the body has to have them. Here is what they are and what they do:

- Cholesterol is a waxy substance that is needed to help digest food and manufacture hormones. It also plays a very important role in the brain and spinal cord.
- Triglycerides are fatty compounds made up of fatty acids and glycerine. Food itself is mostly made up of triglycerides in stored form. Triglycerides are broken down by the body and used for energy.

If you have high blood pressure, the importance of these lipids translates to their level in your blood, a level determined by simple lab tests. Statistics show that your chances of suffering a stroke or heart attack increase if the cholesterol level in your blood is high. Most studies have at least tended to support the idea that there is a link between high triglycerides and coronary artery disease.

Cholesterol Control

For a hypertensive less than sixty-five years of age, the ideal cholesterol level is around 200 to 240 (on an arbitrary scale of measurement), although the ideal varies among doctors.

Cholesterol is found only in animal products. You will find a great deal of cholesterol in:

- egg yolks
- liver
- processed lunch meats
- shrimp, oysters, clams, and scallops

Dairy products are sources of cholesterol, too. Fish and poultry contain cholesterol but are lower in that substance than red meats.

In general, foods that are high in *saturated fats* should be avoided by anyone concerned with cholesterol. A saturated fat usually is solid at room temperature (marbling on a steak). An *unsaturated fat* is usually liquid at room temperature, such as vegetable oil.

Polyunsaturated fats are a kind of unsaturated fat, and are better for cholesterol reduction than *monounsaturated fats*. Examples of polyunsaturated fats are safflower oil, corn oil, soybean oil, and sesame oil. Typical monounsaturated fats include olive oil and peanut oil.

Cholesterol cannot float around the body on its own. It must be attached to a carrier. It can be carried by either a *high-density lipoprotein* (HDL) or a *low-density lipoprotein* (LDL). Most researchers now feel that the proportion of these carriers is what is important. It has been shown that people with high levels of HDL have fewer heart attacks than people with low levels of HDL. Therefore, low levels of HDL are a bad sign.

Smoking gives people much lower levels of HDL. Exercise promotes a higher level of HDL.

In terms of dietary intake and the HDL, it has been shown that high levels of saturated fats increase the LDLs but not the HDLs.

Reducing your dietary intake of cholesterol probably will lower your blood cholesterol level, but not always. To cut back on cholesterol:

1. Reduce your intake of animal products, especially egg yolks and organ meats. With regard to eggs, consult your doctor as to how many, if any, he or she feels you should consume.
2. Use low-fat dairy products.
3. Eat poultry and fish in preference to red meat.
4. If desired by you or suggested by your doctor, undertake a formal cholesterol-control diet. A sample is presented in Appendix C. Your physician will want to monitor your blood cholesterol levels about every three to six months or so. If your high cholesterol levels are the fault of your body's overproduction, rather than your diet, there are a variety of cholesterol-lowering drugs that your doctor may elect to prescribe.

Triglyceride Control

There is no conclusive guide to proper blood triglyceride levels, but your doctor will probably want your reading to be in the range of 200 to 250 (again, on that arbitrary scale of measurement).

A low-calorie diet will usually lower triglycerides. In addition, here are some steps you can take:

1. Stay on a diet low in sweets and saturated fats.
2. Choose foods high in fiber and low in calories, such as vegetables.
3. Monitor your sugar intake carefully. All sugars—table sugars, dextrose, sucrose, fructose, corn syrup, honey, etc.—raise triglyceride levels.
4. Take it easy on your alcohol consumption.
5. Trim fat from your meat, and skin from your chicken. Favor fish, chicken, and turkey over red meat.

Other Dietary Factors

There is a body of evidence that indicates that calcium and blood pressure are somehow related—that low intake of calcium may promote high blood pressure.

As lawyers are fond of saying, the evidence at this point is purely circumstantial. Such data may prove quite meaningful in the future, but at this point it is not prudent to prescribe calcium as a cure to hypertension.

However, maintaining an adequate level of calcium is important for many reasons, including but not limited to prevention of osteoporosis, a degeneration of the bones common in elderly people, especially elderly women.

You certainly can get adequate calcium from your diet, especially from milk and cheese, but those who avoid dairy products because of cholesterol content, or those who cannot tolerate or simply do not like calcium-rich foods, can put themselves at risk for a calcium deficiency.

In order to take in an adequate level of calcium each day (about 800 to 1,200 milligrams), many people take calcium supplements. An example is Oscal, which provides 1,000 mg of calcium in a two-tablet dose. Ask your doctor for additional information on the type of supplementation that is right for you. An adequate calcium intake may or may not prevent hypertension, but we know it will help keep your bones strong throughout your life.

You can get some calcium from nondairy sources such as beans, broccoli, kale, spinach, and collard greens.

Some preliminary evidence indicates that dietary fiber plays a role in lowering blood pressure. Again, the present evidence is inconclusive but we do know that a reasonably high level of dietary fiber is good for just about everyone's digestive system. Why not play it safe and increase your intake of whole grains and fresh vegetables and fruits?

There are certain indications that a vegetarian diet can reduce blood pressure in ways unrelated to sodium intake, potassium level, and body weight. This is a promising area that merits further exploration, but we cannot conclude at this point that a strict vegetarian diet will cure hypertension.

We do know that caffeine can increase blood pressure, so avoid excess consumption.

Another point to consider is food-drug interaction. One particularly important interaction concerns monoamine oxidase inhibitors, known as MAO inhibitors, which are drugs used to treat depression. Typical examples are Nardil and Parnate. Such drugs are used only with caution and with careful monitoring in patients with existing high blood pressure.

MAO inhibitors can cause a steep rise in BP when they interact with certain foods (those that have a high concentration of tryptamine-containing substances or tyramine), such as beer, wine, broad beans, aged cheeses, pickled herring, salami, sour cream, liver, and yeast extract. MAO inhibitors should not be taken with caffeine, chocolate, or certain drugs (those known as sympathomimetic drugs), such as methyldopa, L-dopa, dopamine, adrenaline, or noradrenaline.

If you have a severe reaction, such as headache, fever, sweating, and/or a severe increase in BP, stop taking the MAO inhibitor, stop eating the food in question, and call your doctor.

We hope that diet and its relation to hypertension is now more clear to you. If nothing else, perhaps this chapter has provided a foundation on which to rebuild your eating habits. As you can see, each section contained some relatively complex material, but that material could— and was—boiled down into some general guidelines.

Following general rules may not solve all your dietary problems, but using your head and eating sensibly can help a great deal. As you gain skill in juggling your sodium levels, lipid intake, and calorie allowances, the whole process will become second nature.

Regular exercise, the topic of Chapter 6, will be an important help to your diet plan and will also provide additional physical and psychological benefits unrelated to your diet. Before considering the role of exercise in controlling hypertension, here are some of the more common questions asked about diets and dieting:

Q: What about "crash diets"? I know they work because I have seen my friends lose a lot of weight on them.

A: If we define a crash diet as a very low calorie diet, the main problem is the fact that your eating habits are not reworked; you are thin, but stuck with the same habits that got you in trouble to begin with. Now, very stringent diets do have a place. Some people have experienced success by going on a crash diet and then remaking their eating habits in an effort to maintain that weight. In any event, avoid fad diets.

Q: What is a fad diet?

A: There is no universally accepted definition, but steer clear of any diet that is unduly one-sided—all bananas, all rice, or other such nonsense. Anything that severely alters the usual proportions of foods in a standard diet (such as a no-carbohydrate diet) can mean trouble.

Q: One common factor in all diet advice for hypertensives is to lower intake of fat. True?

A: Good advice for just about anyone. American diets are lopsided in terms of consumption of fats and proteins. As a general rule, you will be better off by increasing carbohydrate intake from grains and vegetables and lowering fat intake. Do not go overboard, because you need a certain amount of fat in the diet, and fat is one of the factors responsible for staving off hunger pangs.

[6]
Lowering
Blood Pressure
through Exercise

This is the era of the jogging suit and the health spa. That, unless you have been totally out of touch with civilization for the last ten years, will come as no surprise.

As with any other subject, exercise can get pretty complicated when you start unearthing the various theories for sharpening sports skills, training methods to heighten endurance, studies on the composition of muscle fibers, and so on. An in-depth discussion of oxygen uptake, for instance, might be helpful to a competitive runner but it just muddies the water for someone who does not exercise regularly and wants to start.

That is why this chapter is short and to the point. Its goal is to clear up some of the mystery surrounding exercise programs and steer you to a simple program you can use and benefit from.

First, definitions of terms. *Aerobic* exercise is the kind we are stressing as most beneficial to hypertensives. Aerobic means "with oxygen" and refers to exercises involving continuous movements, designed to increase oxygen consumption and improve the functioning of the cardiovascular system. *Anaerobic* means lack of oxygen, and refers to movements of brief intensity where there is not a steady and adequate supply of oxygen to the muscles.

Running, jogging, cross-country skiing, jumping rope, bicycling, and vigorous calisthenics involving large muscle groups are examples of aerobic exercise. Anaerobic exercises include weight lifting and stop-and-start sports such as tennis and racquetball.

Both aerobic and anaerobic exercises have their particular uses. Aerobic exercise is far better suited to improving the condition of your cardiovascular system than is anaerobic exercise. Anaerobic movements such as weight lifting, on the other hand, are superior for developing muscle strength and size.

From the standpoint of dealing with hypertension, aerobic exercise

119

should be the mainstay of your program. You will want to engage in continuous, vigorous movements involving the major muscle groups for a period of between twelve to fifteen minutes every day or every other day.

The secret, if you want to call it that, is *consistency*. This cannot be stressed enough, and is backed up by virtually everyone knowledgeable about the exercise process. Sticking to your program over a long period of time is what produces the results—not a murderous two hours once every ten days or so.

In summary, consistent aerobic exercise is what seems to reduce blood pressure most efficiently.

Now, some other terms commonly used are *isometric* and *isotonic*. Isometric basically means that there is no appreciable movement in muscle mass; an exercise where you clasp your hands together and contract your arm muscles is isometric. An isotonic exercise is a movement where there is a great deal of motion of the muscle groups, such as when you perform "jumping jacks." In general, isotonic exercises are better for lowering blood pressure than are isometric movements.

What Exercise Will and Will Not Do for You

In terms of reducing blood pressure, the most popular current theory holds that continued and consistent exercise results in a long-term dilation, or opening up, of the blood vessels. If true, this certainly is the ideal effect for most hypertensives! Blood pressure is automatically reduced by lowering the resistance in the arteries, the same way in which a large hose reduces the pressure of the water flowing within.

Another current theory postulates that since exercise lowers the resting heart rate (a conditioning effect brought on by strengthening the heart muscle), the reduction in baseline heart rate lowers total blood pressure. The heart simply does not keep jamming fluid through the arteries so rapidly.

Both theories are probably true to various extents depending upon the patients and the situations involved.

A review of the latest research findings does substantiate the belief that exercise can lower blood pressure. In fact, about 80 to 90 percent of such studies indicate that there sometimes is a significant reduction. The reduction in these studies ranges from 2 and 10 mm Hg systolic and diastolic to as much as 20 and 25 mm Hg. However, it is important to note again that these studies have been difficult to control in the scientific sense because of all the complicating variables involved in studying patients with hypertension.

But it certainly is fair to conclude that high blood pressure is reduced by exercise to some degree, depending on the individual. Also, it seems clear that the reductions are not related directly to body weight, since some studies have shown no reduction in weight after an exercise program but have shown a reduction in blood pressure.

That is what exercise can do. What it cannot do is replace drug treatment in severly hypertensive patients. It also cannot magically burn off body weight.

There are many patients who exercise regularly and routinely but after their workouts go to the neighborhood bar where they eat and drink for the next four hours. To put this situation in perspective, look at the figures in Table 3. If you entertain notions of ridding your body of a cheeseburger, fries, and milk shake (1,200 calories) by running off the calories while playing tennis (about 400 calories an hour), it will be painfully obvious that the mouth can always outdistance the feet.

Exercise will not undo the effects of smoking or excess alcohol consumption. Also, exercise will not cure the problems brought on by excess weight if you keep that extra weight.

Getting Started

There is no question that you should consult your doctor before starting an exercise program. This warning is repeated often enough to be something of a cliché, but it is very important. Certain underlying diseases or medications you are taking may preclude some forms of exercise.

An exercise stress test may also be indicated if you are over age forty and/or have significant heart disease. Often heart disease is silent until the onset of exercise or some other factor that increases the heart rate. That increase may be just enough to tip your heart into a state of

Table 3. Calories Expended for Various Activities

Resting, Standing and Walking

	calories per minute		calories per minute
Resting in bed	1.2	Kneeling	1.4
Sitting	1.4	Squatting	2.2
Sitting, reading	1.4	Walking, indoors	3.4
Sitting, eating	1.6	Walking, outdoors	6.1
Sitting, playing cards	1.7	Walking, downstairs	7.6
Standing	1.6	Walking, upstairs	20.0
Standing, light activity	2.8	Standing, showering	3.7

Working Around the Home

Washing clothes	2.9	Mopping floors	5.3
Hanging laundry	4.7	Sweeping floors	1.7
Bringing in laundry	3.2	Scrubbing floors	6.0
Machine sewing	1.5	Shaking carpets	6.4
Ironing clothes	4.2	Peeling vegetables	2.9
Making beds	5.3	Stirring, mixing foods	3.0

Do it yourself

Sawing wood	6.9	Pushing wheelbarrow	5.2
Planing wood	8.6	Chopping wood	4.9
Carrying tools	3.6	Stacking wood	6.1
Shovelling	7.1	Drilling	7.0

Sports and hobbies

Jogging	up to 17.0	Badminton	2.8
Basketball	8.6	Rowing	8.0
Ping pong	4.8	Sailing	2.6
Swimming	12.1	Playing Pool	3.0
Golfing	5.5	Dancing	4.0
Tennis	7.0	Horseback riding	3.0
Bowling	8.1	Cycling	8.0

Reprinted by permission of Pennwalt Prescription Division, Rochester, N.Y.

irregular beating or into a full-fledged heart attack.

You will want to start with a *simple* program. Simplicity and patience are the two primary virtues for an exerciser. Complicated programs have the effect of reducing your chances of continuing. And overly stressful programs—programs where you try to accomplish too much too soon—have the effect of discouraging participants and possibly harming them.

The best kind of exercise program for many hypertensives is one that

Figure 8. Six Warm-Up Exercises
Your objective is to do all these exercises the number of times indicated, without resting between exercises. Your best bet is to begin with five repetitions and work your way up to the goal for each.

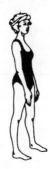 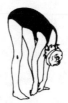

1. Bend and Stretch

Starting position: Stand erect, feet shoulder-width apart.
Action: Count 1. Bend trunk forward and down, flexing knees. Stretch gently in
  attempt to touch fingers to toes or floor. Count 2. Return to starting position.
Goal: 10 times
Note: Do slowly, stretch and relax at intervals rather than in rhythm.

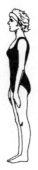 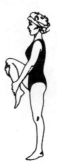

2. Knee Lift

Starting position: Stand erect, feet together, arms at sides.
Action: Count 1. Raise left knee as high as possible, grasping leg with hands and
  pulling knee against body while keeping back straight. Count 2. Lower to starting
  position. Counts 3 and 4. Repeat with right knee.
Goal: 10 left, 10 right

Exercises courtesy of the President's Council on Physical Fitness.

Figure 8, *continued*

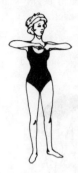 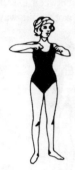

3. Wing Stretcher

Starting position: Stand erect, elbows at shoulder height, fists clenched in front of chest.

Action: Count 1. Thrust elbows backward vigorously without arching back. Keep head erect, elbows at shoulder height. Count 2. Return to starting position.

Goal: 20 times

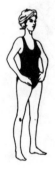 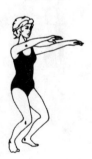

4. Half Knee Bend

Starting position: Stand erect, hands on hips.

Action: Count 1. Bend knees halfway while extending arms forward, palms down. Count 2. Return to starting position.

Goal: 10 times

Figure 8, *continued*

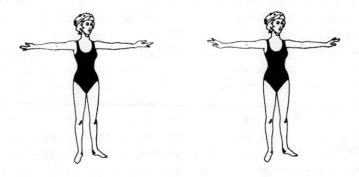

5. Arm Circles

Starting position: Stand erect, arms extended sideward at shoulder height, palms up.
Action: Make small circles backward with hands. Keep head erect. Do 15 backward
circles. Reverse. Turn palms down and do 15 small circles forward.
Goal: 15 each way

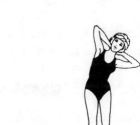
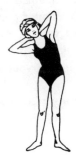

6. Body Bender

Starting position: Stand, feet shoulder-width apart, hands behind neck, fingers
interlaced.
Action: Count 1. Bend trunk sideward to left as far as possible, keeping hands behind
neck. Count 2. Return to starting position. Counts 3 and 4. Repeat to the right.
Goal: 10 left, 10 right

can be done on a regular basis, does not require expensive equipment, and can be done in the privacy of the home.

Outdoor types can pursue vigorous walking or (on the advise of their doctor) jogging, bicycling, or similar sports. However, those of us who live in the Northeast know all too well that severe weather is a powerful deterrent to outdoor activity, and in fact snowy roads can be dangerous to walk or jog on. For people in this situation, treadmills, stationary bicycles, or rowing machines are reasonable alternatives.

Our most immediate recommendation is that you start with a program of simple calisthenics such as those pictured in Figure 8. Calisthenics have the advantage of being easily practiced at home in comfortable clothes (your underwear will do just fine).

A Simple Way to Gauge Intensity Level

Regardless of what type of exercise you choose, the ultimate goal (for the purposes of reducing blood pressure) is to get the heart pumping and the oxygen circulating at a level that is not overly strenuous but provides enough stress for conditioning. You can do this by monitoring your pulse rate. If you do not know how to take your pulse and blood pressure, it is explained in Chapter 10.

You want to monitor pulse rate during the exercise and adjust your exercise so that your pulse rate stays at a certain percentage of your *predicted maximum heart rate*. Your predicted maximum heart rate is calculated by taking your age and subtracting it from 220 beats per minute.

If you are forty years old, your predicted maximum heart rate will be:

$$\begin{array}{r} 220 \text{ beats per minute} \\ - \quad 40 \text{ years of age} \\ \hline = 180 \text{ beats per minute} \end{array}$$

When you are starting out, you will want to keep your pulse at about 60 percent of your predicted maximum heart rate. Using the example above, then:

$$\begin{array}{l} 60 \text{ percent of } 180 \text{ beats per minute} \\ = 108 \text{ beats per minute} \end{array}$$

Your *target rate* is 108 beats per minute.

Any exercise that keeps your heart rate up to around 108 beats per minute (the target rate in this example) for 12 to 20 minutes or so is doing the job.

As you progress and gain fitness, you will want to work up to a level where your target rate is about 75 percent of your predicted maximum heart rate. If you are very healthy, and your doctor agrees, you can eventually work up to 80 or 85 percent.

Remember, take your pulse during exercise and adjust the exercise accordingly to raise or lower your pulse to keep at your target rate. Some people prefer to take their pulse in the side of the neck during exercise, but you can conveniently find your wrist pulse during activity with a little practice. A helpful trick for monitoring exercising pulse levels: Take your pulse for six seconds and add a zero. This gives a reasonably accurate reading of your per-minute pulse rate during periods of activity.

Remember, keep at it. Decide what time of day will be most convenient and religiously stick to your exercise schedule. It can be helpful to monitor your blood pressure before, during, and after exercise and report the results to your doctor. Keep a long-term record of blood pressure, and ask for your doctor's assistance in monitoring your program. Above all, be consistent. This point just cannot be stressed enough.

If you do stay on your program, you can expect to look better, feel better, and be better physically. The results may not appear soon, but results *will* come, given time.

As we will see in the next chapter, exercise also plays a role in reducing the amount of stress we feel. First, some questions and answers dealing with exercise and its role in controlling hypertension:

Q: What about cholesterol and triglyceride levels? Does exercise have an effect on those levels?

A: Yes. Almost all studies on man have shown that there is a direct relationship between exercise and triglyceride levels. The more exercise, the lower the levels (within limits, of course). But when exercise is stopped, triglyceride levels increase—usually within a week.

The effects on cholesterol are somewhat variable. There is an increase in HDLs, which, as was explained in the previous chapter, is a good sign.

Q: I am basically interested in losing weight. But if you look at the amount of calories consumed by exercise, it hardly seems worth it in terms of weight loss. True?

A: If you mean that you cannot reasonably expect to "run off" a big meal, quite true. However, exercise helps many people diet by reducing their hunger level (although this does not work for everyone). Also, there is good evidence that exercise raises your entire metabolism level throughout the day, meaning a further increase in calories burned. Another benefit is that exercise helps you look better by improving body proportions, thus giving further incentive to diet.

Q: I have heard that weight lifting raises blood pressure levels. Would this be dangerous to me, since I already have high blood pressure?

A: Weight lifting is primarily an anaerobic exercise, although fast, high-repetition movements with light weights will have an aerobic effect. As such, most weight training does not play a role in lowering blood pressure. If you overdo it (grunt and groan with heavy weights), you may actually raise your blood pressure, so very heavy lifting is not recommended. Strictly anaerobic and strictly isometric exercises are to be avoided since they may raise blood pressure.

[7]
Lowering
Blood Pressure through
Stress Reduction

Can a state of relaxation lower blood pressure? Before presenting any conclusions, let's take an overview of the body's nervous system and how it relates to stress. In the case of stress reduction, understanding *why* it happens is just as important as understanding how to do it.

The nervous system receives impulses and information from outside the body and directs the activities of the body as a whole. It is divided into the *central* nervous system and the *peripheral* nervous system.

The central nervous system is the brain and spinal cord, the central computer for the whole works. The peripheral system is made up of two parts. One is the system of nerves governed by the brain and spinal cord; these carry information back and forth to the various muscles of the body and to the areas that give us senses, such as the sense of touch.

Essential to stress control is an understanding of the functioning of the other part of the peripheral nervous system, the *autonomic* system, which controls internal organs such as the heart and lungs. It used to be thought that this autonomic system functioned on a completely unconscious level, that is, totally separated from the conscious operation of the brain. Another way to phrase it is that it used to be felt that the conscious operations of the brain had no control over the unconscious operations.

Recent investigations have proven that this is not true. But if blood pressure is an autonomic function (which it is), how can it be controlled by the conscious, thinking brain?

Similar examples exist all through the body. The gastrointestinal tract, for instance, shows how the conscious mind has control over the unconscious. There is a common disease called irritable bowel syndrome or spastic colitis, a disease that causes a hyperactive or spastic bowel and leads to diarrhea when the patient is under stress. *Stress*—perhaps related to a fight with a spouse or to an upcoming final exam, each an event we are dealing with on a conscious level—takes control of the unconscious functioning of the bowel.

There are many other examples of how the conscious mind can, to a certain extent, control the unconscious. One particularly striking type of case is that of a patient given a placebo (a pill containing no effective ingredients) and told that the pill will control his blood pressure. It often *does* lower blood pressure, just because the patient expects it to.

So, depending upon the root cause of your hypertension, your conscious mind may be able to exert some degree of control over the unconscious factors that raise your blood pressure. This is an important point, because if you have a hypertension that is purely related to excess fluid retention, it seems clear that stress reduction will have, if anything, a minimal impact. But essential hypertension that is more of a vasoconstrictive nature can often be altered by psychological maneuvers. This, in fact, was shown more than fifty years ago by a researcher named Edmund Jacobson, who documented that progressive relaxation could result in lower BP.

Such observations led to an abundance of behavior modification techniques to lower blood pressure, including various relaxation therapies and environmental manipulations. Many, but not all, of these techniques have proven effective to a certain degree. The failures probably relate to the etiologies (root causes) of the hypertension cases studied. As discussed above, not all hypertensives will respond to psychological maneuvers. In point of fact, not all hypertensives respond equally well to drugs either. While a diuretic is quite effective for a patient's volume-dependent hypertension, it may not reduce blood pressure at all if used in a case where the patient's hypertension is purely vasoconstrictive. If you follow this to its logical conclusion, you will see why diuretics are only minimally effective in controlling some cases of hypertension yet highly effective in others. The same is true about stress control.

This is a long and rather wordy attempt to convince you that psychological measures really can work under the right circumstances. Evidence that seemingly debunks the effectiveness of stress control does not fully take into account the kind of sampling and testing error noted above.

Stress—What It Is

A scientific definition of stress is: "The sum of all nonspecific phenomena elicited by adverse external influences, including damage and defense." To rephrase that in everyday English, stress basically refers to the effect of all outside forces on your body, whether they be psychological or physical, and the body's resultant change due to those forces.

We are under stress every day of our lives, even during sleep (some dreams are stressful). And, as we know, stress has positive and negative components. On the plus side of the ledger is the fact that stress elevates our blood pressure and speeds up body functions so that we can be more aware and alert when our car starts skidding on a patch of ice, or when unexpected noises are heard downstairs at 3 A.M. In the more primitive applications of stress, we would be prepared for a physical confrontation or to run for our lives. In these cases, stress has been responsible for saving many lives.

But sometimes the stress reaction goes too far. Skidding on the ice can sometimes precipitate a heart attack or stroke or severely elevated blood pressure, especially in an elderly patient. A younger patient might easily adapt until the situation returned to normal, but the stress itself is damaging to that person with cardiovascular disease.

In other words, the stress reaction lasts for inappropriate time frames. When a person gets out of a stressful situation, the autonomic nervous system normally gears down. The action of the autonomic nervous system cuts back, the pulse and BP return to normal, and the body calms itself. But for some people, the stress persists.

In addition, it is clear that many individuals differ in the way they respond to life in general and stress specifically. While some need a great deal of stimulation to feel stress, some react to minimal stimulation. Those people are stress reactors in the same sense that folks who cannot tolerate salt are sodium reactors. A little does a lot of damage.

But an interesting phenomenon can occur in the individual under stress. The noise in the cellar can certainly be frightening—so frightening that your body automatically revs up the stress reaction. But a typical *conscious* reaction might be: "Wait a minute. This is a safe neighborhood and there hasn't been a burglary as long as I've lived here. And even if there were somebody downstairs, the cellar door is locked so he can't get upstairs. Anyway, it's probably the cat after mice again."

Although the example might seem mundane, what has happened is an instance of the conscious mind seizing control of the unconscious. Conscious reasoning slowed down the unconscious stress reaction.

Over the past thirty to forty years, psychiatrists, other physicians, and psychologists have moved with increasing vigor in the effort to find ways to reduce stress. At present, there are many techniques that have been developed and have been proven effective to varying degress in the reduction of stress and resultant lowering of blood pressure.

Regardless of the individual method practiced, the first step usually involves identifying where the stress in your life is. Is it at home? Work? In your social life? Your family doctor, who can measure your physiolgic response to stress and also should be aware of the stress forces in your life, is in a good position to identify the stress and get you started on stress reduction.

Your family doctor also will be able to recommend available resources within your community. For example, your doctor may know of a center that offers access to biofeedback equipment. This can be extremely valuable to a stressful hypertensive.

Relaxation Therapy

Biofeedback stems from two words that mean sending information back to yourself, information that has something to do with biological function. In this particular setting, the idea behind the technique is to learn to lower your blood pressure through various relaxation methods, continually monitoring to gain information on what actions lower blood pressure, so that blood pressure can be lowered even further. The sensations of the activity that lowered tension and blood pressure are reinforced and form a closed loop. An example of this would be a visual or sound recording that varies in intensity with the degree of BP—the higher the BP, the brighter the light or the louder the sound. The subject would attempt to lower the BP by progressive relaxation, and would reinforce success by observing the lowering of visual or auditory levels of the recording.

A technique such as this has to be taught, and special equipment is needed. It has been shown effective in lowering blood pressure, and published studies on biofeedback have shown a 10 to 15 mm Hg reduction of blood pressure.

The benefit-to-risk ratio is extraordinarily good. There are no present contraindications for biofeedback.

One reason put forth as to the success of biofeedback is that the subject, in an effort to lower overall tension, relaxes the muscular-skeletal system. This relaxation itself may be the primary factor in BP reduction.

Utilization of relaxation methods can be practiced without specialized equipment and, in many cases, without formal instruction.

People in Eastern cultures have demonstrated unusual control of their autonomic nervous systems through the use of yoga, which in its simplest form is a method of relaxation. In addition to yoga, relaxation methods include transcendental meditation, Zen meditation, hypnotic meditation, autogenic training, the "relaxation response" outlined by Dr. Herbert Benson, and the Jacobsonian progressive relaxation technique.

Your physician may be able to provide information on where you can receive instruction in the more formalized relaxation therapies. Another good place to start is the local YMCA or YWCA, which may offer related instructions.

Meditation in its simplest form can involve nothing more than sitting quietly, eyes closed, and emptying your mind of all thought; sometimes, meditators use a chant—a word called a mantra—to help in the effort to eliminate distractions. You may find success with meditation of your own making: sitting quietly for fifteen minutes or so each day, feeling the slow, steady breaths enter and leave your body, driving distraction from your brain. While you certainly might benefit from instruction in more formalized meditation practices, the one described in the few sentences above works well for many people.

Hypnosis has worked well as a form of relaxation therapy, but it requires that a technique be taught and learned. Once the technique is mastered, the patient can regularly practice self-hypnosis and reduce blood pressure. Again, it appears that the physical relaxation of the musculoskeletal system may be the underlying reason for pressure reduction.

Of all the relaxation therapies mentioned, we feel that the simplest and most effective is the Jacobsonian progressive relaxation technique, which was originally proposed in a book written in 1929. The book, *Progressive Relaxation*, discussed techniques of relaxation and the effect on the nervous system, including blood pressure.

Dr. Jacobson, in his research, was truly fifty years ahead of his time. He was the first to realize how important the muscular system was, relative to the nervous system. In his book, Dr. Jacobson described how the nervous system could be controlled in part by relaxation of the musculoskeletal system.

His first observations may be very close to the truth of how these techniques lower blood pressure. In the past few years, we have seen that true relaxation of major skeletal muscle groups does lower blood pressure.

We will boil down approximately three hundred pages of Dr. Jacobson's book and tell you how to use progressive relaxation to lower blood pressure:

1. You must have a heightened awareness of the structure of your skeletal musculature, which includes the major muscle groups in the body. You must be aware of whether these muscle groups are tense (contracted) or relaxed (flaccid). Your goal is to learn a method of relaxation that carries no effort. You will, in effect, be feeding relaxation impulses to the muscles.

2. Start building this awareness with your biceps, the major muscle group on the inside of the upper arm. The biceps are responsible for bringing the lower arm upward when the arm bends at the elbow. Contract the biceps forcefully. See how the tone of the muscle changes when it is contracted. Sense its structure under a state of tension. Feel it with your free hand—note the bumps and ridges and the overall tension in the muscle. Now, relax the biceps. Note all the factors above when the biceps is in a relaxed, flaccid state.

3. Lie down in a quiet room and close your eyes. Relax that biceps by sending imaginary relaxation impulses to it. If you sense it tightening up, keep your eyes closed and send more of those relaxation impulses.

4. Now contract the biceps on the other arm. By now, you should be able to do it without moving the arm. Just tighten the biceps. Relax the biceps. Tighten the biceps again. Relax again. Continue feeding those relaxation impulses to the biceps until the muscle group is totally relaxed.

5. Relax all muscle groups in the same manner. You can do it in any order you like, but one easy way is to start with the calf muscles, work up to the front and back of the thigh, the buttocks, the abdominal muscles, the lower and upper back, chest, shoulders, and arms. Follow the general guideline in point 4 but experiment and do what works for you. After a little practice, you can extend your relaxation to smaller muscle groups, such as the eyes and face.

This technique is readily learned and easily used. In experimental trials, it has been responsible for a drop in blood pressures of as much as 20 mm Hg systolic and 15 mm Hg diastolic. One study showed the average to be 4 to 6 mm Hg systolic and 2 to 4 mm Hg diastolic.

If you learn to monitor your own blood pressure (Chapter 10), you will be able to get some idea of the success of your efforts.

Environmental Changes

Any physician will confirm for you that some of the most dramatic changes in blood pressure come about from a change in the patient's environment. Leaving a high-pressure job, for example, can sometimes produce effects as startling as the most powerful pharmacological interventions.

Doctors have something of a slang term for this: an "environectomy." The ending -ectomy means removal, as in appendectomy. Removing the environment itself—the environectomy—is often the only cure for some cases of hypertension.

The environectomy effect is seen every day at the hospital. A typical scenario involves a patient who comes to the hospital with a laceration stemming from catching his finger in a car door. The finger is sutured with no degree of difficulty, but the patient is admitted for observation because his blood pressure is 220/110. Lo and behold, the doctor on rounds the next morning finds that blood pressure has fallen to 130/80 and the patient feels perfectly normal. The drop in BP is due to the alleviation of stress.

This situation is sometimes carried a bit farther when a hypertensive work-up is done in the hospital. The patient was removed from, let's say, an abusive spouse during the hospital stay and the hypertension disappeared. So the work-up done in the safe, sheltered environment of the hospital did not detect the hypertension because the patient had undergone a temporary environectomy. Similar situations have been shown to be responsible for very large reductions in blood pressure, reductions that continued as long as the patient was hospitalized.

Obviously, we can't all check into the hospital every time things get rough. But we can change certain factors in our environment. If the situation is intolerable, you just may have to leave it. Instead of seeking temporary refuge from an abusive spouse, for example, you may have to pack your bags and leave for good or at least find some other remediation for the situation. A high-stress situation on the job may be solved only with your resignation.

These are not easy choices, but they may have to be a part of your own method for beating stress.

Your Personal Stress Reduction Plan

With the exception of the Jacobsonian technique, we have so far talked in abstract terms. Now we will get down to specifics.

What can you do to control stress in your life and in turn possibly lower your blood pressure?

The first step is to think of yourself in terms of being Number One. This may sound simplistic, but it means a lot. In office practice, physicians frequently see external control and manipulations of a patient elevate blood pressure to striking and frightening heights. It is essential that you resolve right now that no one in the world has the right to kill you with a stroke by elevating your blood pressure.

Nagging or harassment can be just as lethal as a gun fired into your brain.

Remember that if you have a stroke, it will be you who pays the consequences—not your boss, not your neighbor, not your friends. Blood pressure control is your responsibility, and you must do whatever needs to be done to lower your pressure.

You can help take care of yourself by paying attention to body vibrations. When your body tells you things are not going well, it often does so by sending you sweating signals, palpitations, headaches, etc. Take immediate steps to combat this situation, either by using your relaxation technique, leaving the environment, or both.

Simply avoiding stressful situations or people can be a big help. All of us have people in our lives who create an uneasy situation for us. In fact, many of these people tend to thrive on making our blood pressure rise. Avoid anyone who makes you feel your blood pressure is going up. Change jobs if you have to. Want it straight from the shoulder? All right: All the money in the world is not worth it if you are confined to a nursing home without the power of speech and unable to move the right side of your body.

Maybe eliminating stress is not simple, but there are some simple things you can do in your life that, if nothing else, will give you a start. Here is a five-point plan for hypertensives:

1. Pick your own technique for lowering stress and use it. We recommend the Jacobsonian method, but anything that works for you is all right. Do your technique daily, and learn to make it a reflex you can call on when you are under stress.

2. Seek some sort of physical outlet to relieve stress. Every boiler has a pressure point, and your job is to make sure you do not exceed yours and blow your top. Play racquetball, hike, play golf; the amount of exercise should parallel the amount of stress you are under.

   Angry at your boss? Visualize his head as your racquetball and blow off some of your steam.

3. Avoid stress in your environment. Do your own surgical environectomies. If trips to your in-laws bother you tremen-

dously, do not go. Explain your feelings to your spouse; tell your spouse the situation is killing you.

4. Listen to your doctor, your family, and your friends. Often, a patient under severe stress is not aware that he or she is in trouble. If your doctor, family, or friends say you look harried or flushed, have your blood pressure checked. Others can often see us more accurately than we perceive ourselves.

5. Of primary importance: Seek help if you need it. Find a psychiatrist, psychologist, pastor, or good friend you can talk to. In many cases a skilled psychotherapist can help you cope with situations you cannot change.

These five steps will not eliminate all stress, but will help alleviate it.

A final point: Some people are skeptical about the role of stress in disease. How, they wonder, can my job as a stockbroker make me sick?

Physicians *know without question* that stress can have devastating effects. Many times a history of a patient who has had a heart attack will turn up an important underlying event or emotional component that triggered it. All doctors have seen young patients suffer acute asthmatic attacks after being severely reprimanded by a parent, or seeing their pet hit by a car, or finding out that their best pal is moving from the neighborhood.

There are plenty of these anecdotes that point out the risks. And in terms of risks, remember that the benefit-risk ratio of stress reduction is wonderful. The risks of reducing stress are very low. The benefits are great.

Before moving on, some typical questions about stress control:

Q: I am a little put off by meditation because it seems so mystical. The business of the magic word seems silly.

A: Actually, the apparent effect of the word, or mantra, is not in the significance of the word itself but just as something on which to concentrate. If you concentrate on the word "one," it helps you avoid thinking about words like "car payment." So there need not be anything quasi-religious or mystical about it. The important thing is to keep the mind blank and take deep, regular breaths.

Q: I would like to exercise but I am not physically able to do things like play racquetball. Is there anything else I can do to fight stress through exercise?

A: Just walking around is helpful. Motion is good for the soul, and not only helps you relax but fights depression as well. There are physical as well as psychological reasons for this.

Q: This all sounds fine, but when I am in a traffic jam, nothing helps.

A: Traffic jams seem to bring out the worst in everyone, and are classic examples of stressful situations that cannot be changed but still cause us to fume. There are many coping mechanisms that might be suggested to you by a psychotherapist, but one simple method is to find something you can do while sitting in a car. If you feel as though you are using the time, rather than being forced to waste time, the stress can be reduced. Some options include dictating notes to a tape recorder, learning a foreign language from a cassette tape, practicing singing or diction lessons, or talking on a CB radio.

[8]
Special
Problems

Hypertension often presents many different faces. High blood pressure in children, for example, requires different treatment than the same problem in a senior citizen. In many cases, the treatment and control of hypertension is complicated by the presence of other diseases. Hereditary factors can complicate treatment and place certain people at greater risk; more blacks than whites, for example, seem to have an inherited tendency toward hypertension. Some hypertensives have resistant types of blood pressure (or are themselves resistant to sticking to their treatment plan) and need special attention and treatment strategies.

This chapter will address these special problems. We will focus on problems of the elderly, people who lose potassium because of their treatment, pregnant hypertensives, patients with concomitant diseases, children, blacks, patients with excessively resistant hypertension, and labile (tremendously variable) hypertension.

We have organized the chapter so that you can locate additional information on a specific problem. However, it is worthwhile to read through the entire chapter—even the parts that do not seem to apply to you directly—because some of the information will probably bear some relevance to your individual case.

Hypertension in Senior Citizens

In the American population over sixty-five years of age, more than 40 percent have high blood pressure. In white senior citizens, the figure is about 40 percent. In blacks, for causes thought to be hereditary, the incidence is much higher, about 55 percent.

If you are a "typical" senior hypertensive, your systolic BP rose through your childhood, and then slowed down in your young adult-hood and into your thirties. But by age forty, it began a sharp rise. Your diastolic BP rose steadily until you hit age sixty, and then the rate of rise tapered off. Eventually your diastolic pressure hit a plateau. So, today you are being treated because you have either just a high systolic pressure (a condition known as isolated systolic hypertension) or both that and a mildly elevated diastolic pressure.

Why did this happen? Well, it relates to the equation doctors use to define blood pressure: cardiac output times peripheral resistance, or, in everyday language,

$$\text{(blood pumped by the heart)} \times \text{(resistance in the arteries)}.$$

As we age, our cardiac output may remain the same or fall, but our peripheral resistance rises because the arteries become more rigid and less able to dilate. As a result, the systolic pressure, the pressure generated as the heart pumps and puts the blood under pressure, will increase.

If you are a senior citizen or plan to be a senior citizen, a knowledge and appreciation of hypertension control is vitally important *because hypertension is the single most important risk factor for cardiovascular disease in older people*.

Seniors and their doctors face some special problems in control of hypertension. First is the fact that an older patient typically responds differently to drug treatment than does a younger patient. This relates to the multiplicity of drugs usually taken by an older patient. Cost is a problem for senior hypertensives, too: some antihypertensive medications are very expensive, and many older Americans have trouble just keeping up with the food, rent, and heat.

Finding the Right Drug

Problem number one facing your doctor is choosing a medication that

    a) is effective in an older patient,
    b) does not interact with other drugs you are taking, and
    c) does not worsen preexisting conditions.

You can be a big help in this effort. First, understand what your doctor wants to accomplish when picking a medication:

- As a general rule, your doctor wants to prescribe a much lower dose of medication for an older patient—about one-half the dosage typically given a healthy young adult.
- Your doctor wants to prescribe a drug you can afford to take.
- Also, your doctor wants a drug that is not taken often or on a complex schedule; he or she knows that you may be taking other drugs, too, and you may be on a complicated drug intake schedule.

The reason for the low dosage is the fact that as we age our nervous systems become more sluggish, and less suppression of that system is needed to control hypertension. Also, your doctor will be conservative with the use of diuretics because many seniors fall victim to potassium washout (explained in the following section).

Cost is on your doctor's mind. The most brilliant diagnosis and treatment does no good if the patient does not take the drug. That is why you should ask for a cheaper alternative if the drugs you are taking are too expensive.

The scheduling difficulty stems from erratic pill taking—a problem typically the fault of both the patient and the doctor. It is not unusual for an elderly patient to be taking from ten to twenty pills a day. If the patient is not vigilant about scheduling and taking the pills, it is easy to get mixed up. One good option is to purchase special pill boxes in which you can place your medications the day or week before; these boxes (available from many drug stores) allow you to arrange your pills in daily dosages.

Doctors can help solve erratic pill taking by making sure that the prescription is written in such a way that specific directions for dosage and taking-times will be printed *on the label of the bottle*. Do not hesitate to ask for this option.

Your doctor can help you maintain a correct schedule of medication by explaining what each pill is, when it should be taken, how it works, and what side effects it may cause. If you do not get such an explanation, ask. If you do not get an adequate explanation, ask again.

The pluses and minuses of your drug will be explained during your consultation. While each drug and each patient will present a different picture, here are some of the general characteristics of drug types used to treat the senior hypertensive:

* * *

Diuretics. Older patients on diuretics often lose too much water when taking diuretics. The problem is made worse if a minor ailment, such as a virus, causes fluid loss that is then compounded by the drug. If you are dehydrated and continue to take a diuretic, you risk a severe drop of blood pressure and possible kidney damage.

Pay attention to your body. You can pick up the symptoms of dehydration long before the critical stage. Look for:

- Dry, sticky mouth
- Lack of mucous or tear production
- Low urine output and brown, thick urine
- Tiredness and lethargy

If you develop these signs, stop taking the diuretic and contact your doctor immediately. Be sure to increase your fluid intake.

Beta blockers. This category of drugs generally has a decreased effectiveness in older patients. Some studies have shown an overall 20 percent rate of response in patients over sixty, as compared to an overall 80 percent rate of response in younger hypertensives. A very important point in favor of their use, however, is a recent study that showed that beta blockers can actually reduce the incidence of a repeat heart attack after a heart attack has been suffered, and reduce sudden death after an initial heart attack. It is our belief that beta blockers should be tried in any patient—particularly a senior citizen—who has presented evidence of a previous heart attack or has a history of sudden death in the family.

Contraindications (reasons not to use) for beta blockers include asthma, chronic obstructive lung disease, peripheral vascular disease, or an instability in the heart rate. If you would like to know why, consult the sections "Hypertension and Heart and Coronary Artery Disease" and "Peripheral Vascular Disease," included later in this chapter under the heading "Concomitant Diseases."

Calcium channel blockers. These agents have been shown effective in the treatment of senior hypertensives. In fact, they have proven to be particularly well suited to an older patient, doing their job while not oversedating the elderly patient's nervous system.

Your doctor will be wary of using nifedipine (Procardia) if you are susceptible to rapid heart beat, angina, or fluid retention. Diltiazem (Cardizem) and verapamil (Calan or Isoptin), on the other hand, can cause a decreased heart rate and can be used quite effectively with a patient suffering too-rapid heartbeat.

One of the biggest drawbacks of calcium channel blockers is their tendency to cause constipation, a major problem for many senior citizens. Calcium channel blockers do *not* interfere with absorption of calcium into the bones, a concern of many senior women.

Centrally acting sympatholytics. These drugs, such as clonidine (Catapres), guanabenz acetate (Wytensin), and methyldopa (Aldomet) are also useful for seniors. Your doctor will warn you to be careful about postural hypotension—a dramatic lowering of blood pressure when you stand up, a problem that could lead to dizziness and falls. Other side effects prevalent in senior citizens include dry mouth, fatigue, oversedation, and depression.

Vasodilators. Drugs such as hydralazine (Apresoline), nitroprusside (Nipride), and minoxidil (Loniten) are used with care in older patients because those medications can cause sodium and fluid retention and often have to be used in conjunction with diuretics.

ACE inhibitors. Not much is known about medications such as captopril (Capoten) and their use with older patients, but it appears that these agents will be quite useful. If your doctor prescribes an ACE inhibitor, he or she will be vigilant in watching for kidney problems (worsening of kidney failure or elevated potassium in blood), which are sometimes aggravated by these drugs.

In *general*, the choice of drugs for treatment of a senior hypertensive begins with diuretics with the addition—if needed—of methyldopa, hydralazine, or clonidine.

As mentioned, dosages will be started low, very low for quite elderly patients.

To Treat or Not to Treat

Perhaps your doctor does not prescribe any drugs at all for your hypertension. Why? There are no simple answers, and the issue is a controversial one.

There are data to support the concept that treatment of mild to moderate hypertension in the elderly decreases illness, and there is very good evidence to show that treatment of hypertension in older patients decreases the death rate. The Framingham study mentioned earlier, a famous scientific project investigating heart disease, examined and followed about five thousand subjects in the community of Framingham, Massachusetts. It showed that treatment of older hypertensive patients basically yielded the same good results as treatment of younger patients.

But the treatment of isolated systolic hypertension (as stated earlier, a common problem of the elderly) has not been so clearly defined. It is generally held—though not conclusively proved—that it is worthwhile to treat isolated systolic hypertension as long as the treatment does not cause troublesome side effects.

In general (if anyone can make a general statement about this complex area), blood pressure in senior citizens should be treated with the goal of reducing the pressure to at least 140/90.

To be frank, some doctors may think that treating an elderly patient's 160/100 BP is worthless, and may in fact cause more problems than it prevents—in other words, treatment would tip the benefit-risk ratio the wrong way.

Well, the jury is still out on this one, and the point cannot be proven either way. For one thing, no scientific evidence shows conclusively at what level treatment should begin. There are few well-defined studies of patients over sixty-five with blood pressure in the mild to moderate range, and you can readily appreciate the reasons:

- It is just about impossible to isolate an elderly population that does not take other drugs.
- It is equally difficult to isolate a similar population that has no other diseases to confuse the results.

• Such a population, if it existed, would probably be difficult to recruit for an intensive experimental study group.

So, what scientists call a "pure" study of mild to moderate hypertension in the elderly has never been done and may never be done. Does this mean that as the years go by we will give up drug treatment because we do not have the data to support the idea? No, we do not think so; once again, the common-sense approach and the clear evaluation of the benefit-risk ratio must be foremost in the doctor's mind. And in general, more seniors with hypertension today are being treated with new-generation drugs that cause fewer risks and side effects.

Some physicians are less familiar with newer treatment programs and are less flexible in their approach. A rigid physician may also tend to stop blood pressure treatment if the patient has side effects, and be less willing to try another approach.

This issue may seem better suited to debate in medical journals (which is indeed what is happening). But it does affect you, and it affects you directly. One of the questions you should ask your doctor— a list follows—deals with this debate over whether or not to treat, or how vigorously to pursue treatment. If you know the facts, you can work with your doctor to make a better decision.

Questions to Ask Your Doctor

To get the most from your medical care, you should ask your doctor the following questions. If you think you might forget, take this book with you.

• *Does my blood pressure really need to be treated?* If the doctor says yes, it is probably because treatment stands a chance of stopping or altering damage that has occurred. If the answer is no, there can be several good reasons. Perhaps you have a conflicting disease that makes treatment too risky or severely limits the choice of drugs available. Another possibility is that you have no end-organ damage and the benefit-risk ratio seems tipped in favor of letting things continue as they are. Similarly, you may have a good family history (no stroke, no heart disease), persuading your doctor that aggressive treatment is not necessary.

- *Will the drug you are prescribing interfere with others that I'm taking?* In order to get an intelligent answer to this question, bring in all the medications you are taking. Put all the bottles in a paper bag and take them to the office with you. The pill your gynecologist may have prescribed could counteract the effects of a pill your family doctor has given you. Ideally, your doctor's answer should be, "No, this drug will not interfere with the effects of the other drugs you are taking."

- *How should I take this medicine?* Get specific instructions on how and when to take the pills. Find out if the drug should be taken on a full or empty stomach. Ask if it can be taken at bedtime.

- *What side effects should I be aware of? Which ones are serious? Do you want me to call if I have problems, and what's a good time to reach you?*

- *How much will this drug cost? Is there a cheaper alternative?* Your doctor should be able to give you a good idea of the cost. If it is too much, the doctor can make a judgment on whether a generic drug would do as well. Some other alternatives exist. Most physicians are given small sample packets of drugs to pass out to patients; ask for a sample packet if you are going on a new and expensive drug. This way, you may avoid wasting $40 on a bottle of nonrefundable pills because they make you sick. Also, investigate the option of buying your drugs in bulk; sometimes you can get a wholesale or near-wholesale price. Retired people should carefully evaluate coinsurance policies. Be sure to calculate drug prices (and possible savings) with an eye toward the annual net cost of the drugs, taking into account the cost of the policy and the amount of the deductible.

Potassium Washout

The loss of potassium is a problem particularly troublesome to senior citizens but it can affect anyone using diuretics. Many people—particularly the elderly—live on a diet deficient in potassium, a metallic element. In general, eating a well-balanced diet rich in fruits will provide enough potassium, but when potassium is low and powerful diuretics wash what is left out of the body, problems can occur.

A lack of potassium may lead to muscle weakness and, in extreme cases, heart rhythm problems that can be fatal.

If you are losing too much potassium, your doctor may elect to place you on a potassium-sparing diuretic. But if potassium-sparing drugs are contraindicated (perhaps due to their high cost), and you cannot get potassium up to adequate levels by reworking your diet, potassium supplementation is warranted.

Supplementing Potassium Intake

Potassium supplementation is something patients frequently ask about but do not completely understand. Doctors, incidentally, are sometimes less than insightful on potassium levels. For example, potassium levels computed in a laboratory are sometimes misleading: There are many patients who have potassium levels on the low side of normal who have no symptoms whatsoever. It is not uncommon for physicians to treat the lab results—and not the patient—by prescribing potassium supplements automatically when the numbers appear low.

But when you *do* have symptoms, such as muscle weakness or spasms, potassium supplementation is in order. And if you are subject to irregular heartbeats and/or are taking the drug digoxin (for a heart problem), your physician will almost certainly prescribe potassium supplementation.

There are a great number of potassium supplements on the market. The cheapest but hardest to take is a liquid—a simple, 10-percent solution of potassium chloride. The most expensive but easiest to swallow are wax-coated tablets that dissolve in the digestive tract.

Here is another area where you can take a direct role in determining the cost of your drug therapy. If you can choke down the potassium solution, and if your doctor agrees that it is right for you, do it. Potassium has a bitter, and—for some people—repulsive taste. Mixing the potassium in orange juice helps a great deal, but some people still find it nauseating.

Pharmaceutical companies have designed many alternatives for hiding the taste of potassium. It has been placed in an effervescent seltzer, in powders, in pills, and in wax tablets. The wax tablets slowly release the potassium so as to avoid stomach upset. Patients with ulcers or very sensitive stomachs should opt for the wax tablets, known to doctors and druggists as *wax enterics* or *wax matrix tablets*.

As the complexity of the potassium-hiding mechanism increases, so does the price of the medication. Do not overlook this factor when you are considering the options. Remember, you are going to be taking perhaps a hundred pills a month, over a thousand pills a year.

Now, another practical point: If you take wax enterics, do not feel cheated when you see what appears to be the same three pills you took yesterday floating in the toilet bowl. The wax skeletons of the pills do not dissolve in the digestive tract. But the medicine does get into your system.

Slow-K was one of the first potassium tablets. (K is the symbol for potassium, and is incorporated into the names of most potassium-containing drugs.) Slow-K contains 8 milliquivalents of potassium; a milliquivalent is a complicated measurement that defines a certain volume but incorporates other measurements as well. Koan-CL, Klotrix, K Tabs, and Micro-K are common potassium-containing tablets, and they contain 10 milliquivalents. Twenty-five milliquivalents is what you will get from the standard dose of the potassium solutions commonly dissolved in orange juice.

It is important to remember that you and your doctor will have to follow symptoms and reactions closely after you begin taking extra potassium. If, for example, your muscle cramps do not disappear after "K level" is brought back to normal, you have some other type of problem.

It is possible to take in too much potassium. The most serious effect of too much potassium occurs when a patient's kidneys do not work well in the first place. When there is too much potassium in a body with normal renal function, the kidneys simply speed up their function and excrete it. But if the kidneys are not up to the job, K levels build up and can interfere with normal heart function, causing slow heart beat or a *heart block*. A heart block is what happens when the electrical impulses the heart uses to trigger itself become jammed, and the beating of the four pumping chambers becomes uncoordinated.

When you take potassium or any other medication, or even vitamins, remember that if a little is good, a lot is not necessarily better.

Blood Pressure and Pregnancy

This is a very special problem because it deals with the health of the mother and the infant. Babies of hypertensive mothers are often small for the gestational age and sometimes very fragile. It is thought that this is due to a diminished flow of blood to the uterus.

In severe cases, hypertension can lead to toxemia in the mother. Toxemia is a general collection of symptoms (what doctors call a "wastebasket diagnosis"), including seizures, coma, swelling, and a high level of protein in the urine.

Hypertension during pregnancy is almost always essential hypertension aggravated by the pregnancy. In some women with borderline hypertension, blood pressure readings can go virtually out of sight during pregnancy, so careful monitoring is important.

Step Zero treatment is often not helpful to a pregnant hypertensive, but she should pay particular attention to weight control, salt reduction, and avoidance of smoking. Diuretics are usually the drugs of choice for this special problem. If thiazide diuretics are not effective, then treatment will proceed with such drugs as beta blockers or methyldopa. These drugs will not harm the baby.

Concomitant Diseases

There are many diseases that go hand in hand with hypertension, for reasons still largely unknown. For example, 15 percent of all hypertensives have angina pectoris (chest pain), 14 percent have diabetes, 13 percent have congestive heart failure, 8 percent have renal impairment, and 7 percent have asthma. The link with some of the concomitant—meaning "going along with"—diseases is understandable (such as the examples of heart and kidney damage shown in Chapter 1), but with others it is still a mystery.

Ailments such as glaucoma, peripheral vascular disease, heart and coronary artery disease, hyperlipidemia (high fats in the blood), gout, and scleroderma (a skin disease) are also frequently found in hypertensives.

It is possible that therapy to control blood pressure could improve some of these conditions, or at least keep further damage from occurring. Keep in mind, though, that in the complex body systems, cause and effect are not always easily distinguishable. Let's look at some major concomitant diseases and see how they relate to hypertension and hypertension control.

Hypertension and Heart and Coronary Artery Disease

As an example of the body's refusal to do things that make sense in theory, let's look at atherosclerosis. While decreasing blood pressure *should* bring about a decrease in death due to atherosclerosis, the results in real life are not what they should be on paper. In other words, there must be some other physiological processes occurring in patients with coronary artery disease, and hypertension is not the entire cause nor the entire cure.

Decreasing cholesterol has definitely been shown to decrease mortality due to coronary artery disease. But if you are being treated for hypertension, your doctor must exercise caution in prescribing such drugs as the thiazide diuretics and/or beta blockers, which may actually increase fat levels in the blood. There is vigorous debate in medical circles as to the long-term effects of thiazides and beta blockers, and that debate is currently unresolved. If you have a history of elevated lipids (blood fats) including cholesterol, be sure your doctor or doctors know about it.

On the other side of the coin is the discovery that beta blockers have been shown to decrease the risk of second heart attacks.

Calcium channel blockers show promise in treatment of patients with hypertension and cornorary artery disease. They act simultaneously to ease angina pains and to lower blood pressure.

Captopril, an ACE inhibitor, has shown promise, too. Runaway functioning of the renin-angiotensin-aldosterone system is a major factor in congestive heart failure, and ACE inhibitors help to regulate this problem.

Diabetes

Diabetes, hypertension, and elevated lipids—in any combination—are *additive* in their cardiovascular risk. Just as some drugs act synergystic-ally to make treatment more effective, so some ailments act in concert to worsen an illness. A diabetic's risk of cardiovascular trouble is very, very high; any influencing (additive) factors must be controlled at all cost.

The problems you and your doctor might encounter include the aggravating effect some drugs have on blood sugar: Thiazide diuretics increase blood sugar and blood fats. A diabetic who is taking antihypertensive agents must monitor his or her blood sugar carefully once drug therapy is started.

There are some agents, such as nonselective beta blockers, that can lower blood sugar and actually blunt the patient's sensitivity to symptoms of that blood sugar drop. One patient who encountered this problem, for example, was placed on beta blockers by a doctor who apparently was not aware of her diabetes. She developed seriously low blood sugar, but all her usual warning signs were blocked. Only the fact that she conscientiously monitored her sugar levels saved her from serious consequences.

Here is the moral of the story, and it applies to more than diabetes: The doctor who diagnoses your diabetes may not be the one who diagnoses your hypertension, or the situation may be reversed. In fact, the specialist or subspecialist who diagnoses or treats any problem may not be aware of your hypertension, or your diabetes, or any other illnesses, so *be sure you mention them.* Our poorly treated diabetic friend in the example above should have mentioned her diabetes to the doctor who prescribed the beta blocker. And, of course, the doctor who wrote the prescription should have found out about her diabetes.

Captopril is emerging as a popular drug for treatment of hypertensive diabetics because it does not appear to affect blood sugar levels.

Renal (Kidney) Disease

In general, your doctor will have to take special precautions with drugs that are excreted by the kidneys. Potassium-sparing agents must be used with care because patients with kidney problems have trouble excreting potassium. In most patients with renal failure, potent loop diuretics are used because they forcefully increase the flow of urine in an impaired kidney, which in most cases is exactly what the doctor ordered.

If you have kidney disease and hypertension, be aware that it is crucial for you and your doctor to control this problem because the two factors can catch you up in a vicious cycle: Kidneys get worse. Blood pressure reflexively gets higher to compensate. Higher BP further damages kidneys, etc.

Asthma and Chronic Lung Disease

Certain beta blockers are not good choices for a patient with asthma or chronic lung disease because the nonselective beta blocking agents can act at the smooth muscle cells in arteries and in the bronchial tree and cause a constriction. That, of course, is exactly what you do not want.

A doctor who knows you have asthma or chronic lung disease will prescribe a drug that is more selective and lowers blood pressure without aggravating breathing problems. Be sure you mention breathing problems to a doctor treating you for any illness.

Gout

This disease is characterized by a high uric acid level in the blood, and is associated with monarticular arthritis, meaning arthritis in one joint only. Some drugs, such as certain beta blockers and thiazide diuretics, have been shown to elevate uric acid level.

If you suffer from gout, or if you have developed goutlike symptoms (pain in a joint, often the big toe), mention the problem to your doctor. Prazosin, captopril, and the calcium channel blockers can all be used safely for individuals with gout.

Peripheral Vascular Disease

Peripheral vascular disease is a name for the narrowing of the medium-sized arteries of the body. A common example is an elderly patient with a history of *intermittent claudication*—pain in the legs during exercise, pain that comes and goes. What happens is that patients have a restriction of the flow of blood to the leg muscles, and those muscles rebel and scream out during exercise.

Your doctor will want to avoid beta blockers if you have peripheral vascular disease.

A special area of peripheral vascular disease is a relatively common ailment called Raynaud's phenomenon. This is a disease of unknown origin that occurs with relative frequency in young adults and elderly patients. It causes a spasm of the arteries in the hands or feet with a concomitant lack of blood to those extremities. Then, the body triggers a subsequent dilation of those blood vessels. The patient experiences white hands or feet when exposed to cold temperatures. The extremities may even turn purple. Be sure to mention any such symptoms to your doctor because unless you are exhibiting symptoms at the time of the examination, even a complete physical will not reveal this condition.

Propranolol may aggravate Raynaud's. Some of the newer calcium channel blocking agents have been shown to help alleviate it.

Depression

About 20 to 25 percent of senior citizens suffer from some degree of depression. Depression can complicate treatment of patients because many antihypertensive agents cause or aggravate depression. The most notable such drugs are reserpine, the centrally acting drugs, and some beta blockers.

Depression does not show up in a physical examination, so make certain you mention it to your doctor *because the wrong drug is going to make a bad situation worse*. From the doctor's standpoint, treatment of a depressed hypertensive may open up a whole new arena of anger and depression with the focus being the doctor and the drug. This makes complying with pill-taking difficult for the patient and diagnosis of the problem difficult for the doctor.

Reserpine is one of the worst depression-aggravators, but some doctors continue to use it in patients who are likely to be depressives.

Incidentally, drugs can also be the indirect cause of some bouts of depression, such as those due to hair growth from minoxidil or sexual impotency from beta blockers.

Thyroid Disease

Both overactive and underactive thyroid function can be associated with hypertension. In hyperthyroidism (too much) there is usually a very rapid heartbeat; hypothyroidism (too little thyroid function) causes a slower heartbeat.

If you are in the hyperthyroid category, your doctor will probably prescribe a beta blocker, which slows down the heart rate. If hypothyroidism is the problem, your doctor will rule out beta blockers in deciding on your treatment.

Hypothyroidism sometimes poses a threat because it is associated with high blood lipid levels.

Hereditary Factors

Possibly the most important part of a medical history is a determination of how your family fared with hypertension over the years. The doctor cannot measure this factor exactly, but it might be the influencing piece of information in the choice of a certain treatment program.

Example: A forty-five-year-old executive has borderline hypertension. His doctor takes a history and finds that the patient's brother is obese and hypertensive, and the patient's father died of a stroke at age fifty.

What should be done? The best option would be very aggressive treatment—and letting the patient know that if he does not shape up, the handwriting is on the wall.

When there is any question of family history, one of the first things the doctor wants to know about is lipid levels, which appear to have a strong hereditary linkage.

A discussion of blood lipids (fats) could occupy a book in itself, but in terms of hypertension it is worth noting—as mentioned earlier—that the two factors are additive in their cardiovascular risk.

Blood lipids are calculated by laboratory tests on blood drawn from the patient. It is essential that you not be under any stress when the blood is drawn, and that you fast for at least eight hours prior to the test. If the lipids are elevated, the test should be repeated two or three times during the course of treatment to determine if the high blood lipids are hereditary in origin.

This is an important point, because hereditary high blood lipids often can not be controlled by diet alone. While many people can lower cholesterol by lowering cholesterol intake (as outlined in Chapter 5), a person with hereditary lipid problems may have a metabolic system that is virtually a cholesterol factory, pumping out excess cholesterol even if the intake of cholesterol is near zero.

If this is the case, the patient is at very high risk for cardiovascular problems, and control is critical.

In terms of heredity, essential hypertension itself, as well as many of the concomitant factors, appears to be passed from generation to generation. Did your father have hypertension? Then you are at greater risk of having it or developing it. Did both parents have hypertension? Then your risk factor is extremely high.

The gene that carries hypertension has not been identified, and many of the hereditary factors are unknown, but common-sense observation and the best available statistics do show a connection. Here is a linkage that is very important to you, the hypertensive, because *other members of your family may be at risk*. Tell your parents, brothers, and sisters, and be sure that your children are screened for hypertension.

This bit of information—combined with some persuasion on your part—can be lifesaving to members of your family.

Hypertension in Children

So does this mean that your children could have hypertension now? Is it realistic to ask the pediatrician to check BPs on your kids? Does hypertension in children cause any lasting harm?

The answers are *yes, yes, and yes.*

If you have hypertension, the probability that your children have it or will have it is extremely high. The overall incidence of childhood hypertension is from 1 to 10 percent of the total population. More and more pediatricians and family doctors are now taking blood pressure measurements; because such measurements are not and have not been universally taken, the true incidence is not known.

Alert your child's doctor to the family's history of hypertension. Ask the doctor to take the youngster's blood pressure. A pediatric blood pressure cuff is used in young children and an adult cuff may give inaccurate readings of blood pressure.

Does an elevated blood pressure in a child cause any lasting harm? You bet it does. High blood pressure causes its effects (in most cases) dependent upon how long the patient has been hypertensive. Therefore, it is in the pediatric population that the doctor has the best chance of halting the damaging effects of blood pressure.

In children, the exact level at which we classify them as hypertensives is not well defined. However, children are usually considered hypertensive if their blood pressure levels are higher than those of 90 percent of the children in their same age group. Once again, the diagnosis is not made until the child's blood pressure has been measured a number of times.

In children, unlike adults, secondary hypertension is a very common diagnosis. Renal diseases are common causes. It stands to reason that a detailed physical exam and laboratory work-up should be undertaken when hypertension is present in children, with a particular emphasis on evaluating renal function.

Treatment of hypertension in children often, then, is related specifically to treating their underlying secondary causes of hypertension.

If the child has essential, chronic hypertension, then treatment similar to the adult stepped-care program is called for. Once again, Step Zero treatment, especially weight loss, is employed first. If there is an inadequate response, then drug management will be instituted, usually using dosages smaller than for adults.

Diuretics are usually not used as a Step One drug on children. Beta blockers are often the drug of choice. Calcium channel blocking agents and ACE inhibitors are also well tolerated by children.

With any treatment, the child's physical and mental growth and development, as well as sexual maturation, must be monitored. Treatment of high blood pressure in children has its special problems, but the long-term rewards are great.

Hypertension in Blacks

Another example of heredity and hypertension is the predisposition of blacks to hypertension. Not only do blacks have significantly increased risks of having high blood pressure; the *effects* of untreated high blood pressure in blacks appear more devastating than for other racial groups. The incidence of hypertension in blacks is double that of whites—but the mortality rates are a staggering fifteen times higher in young black males as compared to young white males. If you are a young black male, you should be very concerned with this statistic.

Physiologically, blacks usually have a good response to diuretics, indicating that a great majority suffer from volume-dependent hypertension. In general, blacks do not respond as well to beta blocker therapy as do whites, probably for the above-cited reason. The remainder of the stepped-care approach is nondiscriminatory and the drugs are used as in the white population.

Unmanageable and Unmanaged Hypertension

True refractory (unmanageable) hypertension is rare. Only 4 or 5 percent of patients cannot be helped. More often, it is the *patient* who is resistant to treatment, rather than the blood pressure.

The most common cause of hypertension that just cannot seem to be brought under control is noncompliance with treatment—in other words, not taking the medication. Another common problem is inappropriate drug treatment, or perhaps drug treatment that is nullified by interaction with other drugs. When blood pressure will not come down, it may also be caused by factors other than essential hypertension: kidney disease, perhaps. This patient gets sent to a specialist.

But let's get back to the fact that the patient's failure to comply with treatment is the biggest factor in blood pressure that refuses to budge. Here are some reasons why patients do not take their medicines properly:

- Lack of money
- "Feeling better"
- Confusion
- Not caring
- Fear of side effects

Lack of money, as addressed earlier in this chapter, can indeed be a problem because of the expense of some antihypertensive agents. "Feeling better" is a terrible reason to stop taking your drugs, because as you are certainly aware by now hypertension usually does not produce symptoms until the damage is done. Confusion and forgetfulness are common to many patients, not just the elderly. Use of pill boxes and getting someone to help in your drug regimen are useful.

Some people just do not have the aptitude to appreciate the scope of the problem and the need to take their medication, and they simply do not care enough to follow a treatment program. Judging from the fact that you have made the effort to read this far, you certainly do not fall into this category.

The final factor is an extremely important one, and deserves some discussion. Even concerned, intelligent patients sometimes slack off on medications because of side effects, fear of side effects, or imaginary side effects.

Part of the problem stems from the fact that informed-consent laws have proven to be a two-edged sword. A physician prescribing an antihypertensive agent may feel obligated to list every major or minor side effect that may occur. Like anything else, a little of this is good but too much is harmful. When the doctor rattles off a laundry list of a hundred side effects, it is no wonder the patient is afraid to take the pills!

We are repeating ourselves, but this is a point worth repeating: The majority of patients can take most of the antihypertensive drugs on the market without unpleasant side effects. But fixating on side effects can *cause* side effects. Patients told that they can expect tiredness often feel tired just because of that prophecy, or blame normal tiredness on the pills. Similar situations occur with impotence, dizziness, and other symptoms.

Your doctor can usually order tests that separate the actual side effects from the psychosomatic ones.

Labile Hypertension

"Labile" means unstable. Everyone's blood pressure is labile to a degree, but in some patients—most notably young adults or middle-aged adults—blood pressure fluctuates tremendously from hour to hour and day to day.

A typical labile hypertensive, if there is such a thing, is an executive who drinks eight cups of coffee a day, does not exercise, runs from meeting to meeting, and has three cocktails at lunch and at dinner. His

BP can vary anywhere from 90/70 to 190/130 within a short period of time, depending on what factors are controlling it.

If you recognize a little of yourself in this portrait, also recognize the fact that your hypertension may be extremely difficult for a physician to diagnose and treat in an office setting. You may, for instance, have been diagnosed as having "office high blood pressure" (caused by the stress of being in a doctor's office) and sent home without treatment. Perhaps this happened to you at a time when the dangers of labile hypertension were not yet fully realized. Today, we know that labile hypertension is indeed dangerous, and that danger is directly related to how high the blood pressure climbs and how often it climbs. Some researchers now feel that the rapid rise itself is just as dangerous as a sustained high blood pressure.

One of the best methods of control for people in this category is home blood pressure monitoring, which is explained in Chapter 10. By learning how to check your blood pressure, you can tell what triggers the peaks. Also, you will see that your BP is indeed high, and this will motivate you to do something about it.

By the way, a labile patient can effectively participate in his or her own treatment by letting the doctor know when BP is high and when it is low. You can—with your doctor's permission—cut back on medication if BP is low over a period of time, or add a half a pill when it starts to climb.

Beta blockers are frequently the drug of choice for this type of individual. Biofeedback and medication are often effective.

Admittedly, dealing with the types of problems explored in this chapter involves a great deal of effort, both from the patient and the doctor. And while such problems may seem complex and difficult, look at the situation from the other point of view: Twenty—or even ten— years ago there would have been very little help available to you. Do not look on your pills and your treatment regimen as the enemies, because they are not. They are tools to increase your life span, and marvelously ingenious tools from a technical point of view.

New advances in hypertension control emerge almost weekly, and the next chapter will detail what is on the horizon. First, three quick questions commonly asked about special problems in hypertension:

Q: The section on hypertension in pregnancy related directly to women, but most material in the book treats men and women the same. Is their hypertension similar?

A: Yes, with one exception. Women have hormonal changes, especially before their periods, that often cause them to retain more fluid. This excess fluid can cause blood pressure to rise.

Q: Is hypertension found more frequently in men or in women?

A: In terms of numbers men have more cases of hypertension. But with more women entering high-pressure positions in business, increases in hypertension in women appear to be a result of this factor.

Q: One of the major points made in the chapter was to inform your doctors of your hypertension. Won't that be insulting to them?

A: No. In fact, a patient who volunteers his or her history is held in high regard by a doctor. While most specialists or subspecialists will make an effort to screen patients for hypertension, sometimes the information gets passed over.

Tell *any* doctor—even if he's treating you for a broken finger—about major diseases, allergies, or drugs.

Along the same lines, this is a good place to mention our belief that you should have *one* family doctor to monitor *all* your drugs and *all* your interaction with specialists. A patient who shuttles from specialist to specialist or clinic to clinic can wind up with a cabinet full of drugs that may not interact well with one another. Regardless of how many different doctors you see, you need a doctor who knows your whole history and entire course of treatment.

[9]
Advances on
the Horizon

One of the reasons this book was written in the first place was to meet the needs of people who tried blood pressure control but were unhappy with the results. Perhaps the medications they took produced unacceptable side effects, or the pill-taking regimen proved too complex. Or possibly the medicines or Step Zero therapy were simply ineffective.

Anyone who is returning to the mainstream of blood pressure control will find that things have changed in the past few years. We are learning more—much more—about the aggravating factors of essential and secondary hypertension. New medicines can zero in on body malfunctions with great accuracy, and physicians are undergoing much more thorough training in the use of aggressive new treatment programs.

The body of knowledge in blood pressure research is expanding tremendously. We have come farther in the last couple of decades than we managed to move in the previous couple of centuries. New theories, medicines, and treatment programs are developed with astounding speed today.

This has many implications for the patient and the doctor. First, things are looking up for hypertensives. The treatment plans are becoming safer, more effective, and easier to follow, and today's problem will probably be answered by tomorrow's research. Second, it is pretty difficult to keep up with all this, even for the doctor—come to think of it, *especially* for the doctor, who has bushels of new research material cross his desk every week.

The rapid advance in blood pressure control also means that new developments will certainly occur between the time we write this book and the time you read it. That is why this chapter forecasts some of the exciting changes ahead.

A few words of explanation: The popular press sometimes reports on medical "breakthroughs" that hold promise but turn out to be total flops. Starting with the first announcement of the breakthrough and well past its eventual debunking, physicians are inundated with requests for the new miracle form of treatment.

The worst-case scenario concerns "cures" for cancer, and the most outlandish stories are usually those reported in supermarket tabloids. But the type of medical coverage you will read in quality publications is not generally sensationalized; the breakthrough may not live up to its promise, and it certainly will not be right for every patient, but usually the treatment will hold some validity. At the very least, it will merit further investigation.

It may surprise you to realize that doctors have a difficult time keeping up with it all. In the field of cancer research, for instance, new treatments appear with such speed that a professional network has been established so doctors can check out reported developments—developments that appear on a daily basis.

Blood pressure research does not capture the attention of the media and the public in the way cancer research does, although you could probably make a case for comparing the relative deadliness of cancer and hypertension. However, new ideas do find their way to the public from time to time.

This preamble is a rather wordy way of telling you not to believe everything you read, but do not discount it, either. And just because your doctor has not heard about it, do not assume it is quackery. Maybe he or she has not gotten to that pile of mail on the corner of the desk. Bringing it up will not hurt. Doctors *do* get irritated at patients who badger them for miracle cures dealing with astrological signs or Mexican mystics. They do not get upset by intelligent queries concerning the latest research. In fact, it is sometimes how they *find out* about the latest research.

Advances in Drug Therapy

The most important step in control of hypertension is finding the exact pharmaceutical key that fits the lock in individual cases. One outgrowth of the lock-and-key research has been the recent development of specialized medical centers that, in a short period of time, can run a patient through a series of tests and diagnose the root causes of hypertension.

It is not too unrealistic to think that in the very near future a patient may be able to visit one of these centers and—after examination of a couple of tubes of urine and blood and possibly an X-ray—have his diagnosis spit out by computer. In fact, in the field of diagnosing hypertensions relating to the kidney, we are coming closer to this type of arrangement: We can measure the exact amount of renin excreted from each kidney and track down whether a kidney is excreting too much renin and driving up the blood pressure. If you have a troublesome problem, it is likely your family doctor—who should know about these centers—will refer you to the closest facility.

Another related development is the use of intravenous (injected directly into a vein) ACE inhibitors. Saralasin is a new drug that, when given intravenously, will usually produce a profound reduction in BP in a patient who has renin-induced hypertension.

The whole renin-angiotensin-aldosterone chain is coming under closer scrutiny by scientists. In fact, we are getting to the point where hormones can be measured precisely in the blood.

Advances in Surgical Treatment

Kidney-related hypertension can now frequently be correctly by the surgeon's scalpel. As explained in Chapter 1, a narrowing of the renal artery can cause elevated renin and runaway hypertension. Surgeons recently developed a technique to insert a balloon into the renal artery and widen the narrowed section by inflating the balloon. It appears that this type of operation will become increasingly common and replace many of the cut-and-sew options now available.

The balloon type of treatment is called angioplasty, and it shows increasing promise in a number of areas, including coronary artery surgery. Within the realm of treating blood pressure, it is safe to say that there are very few events as pleasing to a doctor and a patient as a totally awake patient undergoing angioplasty and seeing his BP drop by fifty points within an hour of the procedure.

If the renal artery is unable to be dilated, an exciting new technique involves replacement of the artery with a plastic tube.

What a Patient Should Know about Drug Development

The rapid rate at which new agents are being tested in the control of hypertension is one of the reasons why blood pressure treatment is so confused and confusing today. But this chaos certainly will result in the eventual introduction of new drugs that will profoundly alter the treatment of hypertensives.

A good example of a drug on the forefront of research is captopril (Capoten). It blocks the formation of renin and stops the cascade of events in the runaway renin-angiotensin-aldosterone syndrome. At present, this is the prototype of drugs in the ACE (angiotensin-converting enzyme) field—but there are many drugs being developed right now that work in the same general fashion. Enalapril (Vasotec) is another. Researchers hope that the new ones will have greater effectiveness and fewer side effects.

Calcium channel blockers are an exciting new category of medications that have been found effective in lowering blood pressure as well as in helping the function of a sick heart. These agents were previously approved by the Food and Drug Administration for treatment of angina, but were given FDA approval for treatment of hypertension only days before the time of this writing. Many doctors prescribed them for hypertension control before the FDA gave this recent approval.

This brings us to a serious problem, since it is an example of the kind of ethical dilemma doctors face regularly. Calcium channel blockers were shown to be effective antihypertensive drugs in Europe, and were approved for treatment of angina in the United States. Still, a physician in the United States was technically breaking standards when prescribing the drug for a hypertensive. Should the patient be given a drug that does not have FDA approval, but has been shown experimentally to be effective in controlling hypertension? Is the doctor ethically and medically responsible for the use of that drug? Will the doctor be liable if the patient has an adverse reaction to the drug? Should the patient *take* such a drug?

There are no easy answers, and very few difficult answers, either. The best a doctor can do is to use his or her knowledge of the drug, its effectiveness, and its side effects, and be sure that it is the best drug available. The doctor and the patient have to consider this in an above-board fashion, with full recognition that the drug has not been FDA-approved and—given the slowness of this type of mechanism—it may not be approved for years.

Captopril is another good example of the problem. Prior to its discovery, doctors did not have a drug that worked effectively in certain cases of congestive heart failure. But despite its widespread use for other conditions, captopril was not FDA approved for this application. Doctors used it anyway; it is not too unusual to have a patient in the waiting room who would not be alive were it not for captopril.

Once again, this is a difficult situation for everyone, and it is not a case of doctors in white hats fighting black-hatted bureaucrats of the FDA. While many physicians feel the system of drug testing and approval is far too cumbersome, there are many good reasons for the extensive testing drugs must undergo.

Protecting the public against quackery is one such justification. Happily, hypertensives are not met with the same kind of crackpot cures that appeal to desperate cancer patients who are fighting for their lives, or arthritis sufferers who live with daily pain. (The unhappy side of this equation is that hypertensives usually do not get too excited about their disease because they fail to realize how dangerous it is.)

Some antihypertensive treatments do border on the old wives' tale category, though. Included are such "treatments" as wearing garlic around the neck. Other medications include herbs and spices, none of which have been scientifically shown to be effective. But since many common drugs used today have been derived from plants, we will keep an open mind and be ready to accept treatments, from whatever source, that can pass scientific muster.

Delivery Systems

One intriguing area, separate from drugs themselves, concerns the systems whereby those drugs are placed into the body. As far as taking pills, new methods of encapsulating the medicine will mean less frequent dosing. In the future, people who now must take four pills a day will probably be able to take one a day or possibly one every other day.

It is well known that patient compliance with treatment increases significantly as the frequency of drug administration decreases. In other words, if you have to take only one pill a day, you are more likely to do so faithfully than if you must take several. The so-called wax matrix tablets promise to release medication into the system very slowly. Therefore, some specific drugs that now must be taken into the system gradually—meaning, say, four pills a day—will be emitted little by little from only one pill.

Ideally, many patients soon will not have to take pills at all. They can simply slap on a patch that releases medication through the skin. A popular clonidine (Catapres) application system, for example, allows once-a-week application of a small patch on various parts of the body. The medicine enters through the skin, and there is twenty-four-hour, minute-by-minute sustained release of the drug. This eliminates the peak-and-valley effect of oral drugs, and obviously has a tremendous advantage from the standpoint of patient compliance.

The patch delivery system was first used for nitroglycerine, and at the time of this writing has been expanded to clonidine and motion-sickness medications. It is likely that this type of delivery system could someday be applied to almost all antihypertensive medications.

Some current research deals with implantation of plastic capsules under the skin. At present, the life span of such capsules is limited, but it is a promising type of delivery system.

On the Horizon

In terms of research into hypertension, as stated earlier, we have come farther in recent decades that in previous centuries. Unfortunately, there are still a thousand years to go.

However, it is safe to say that a patient who has not had experience with blood pressure control in the previous ten years will be considerably more satisfied by what is available today.

You can find out more about medical developments by reading quality publications—the medicine sections of national news magazines, for example. If you are interested in additional literature on items related to blood pressure, heart disease, or the cardiovascular system, you can contact various public and private agencies, such as:

The National Heart, Lung and Blood Institutes of the
National Institutes of Health
Bethesda, MD 20205

The American Heart Association
7320 Greenville Avenue
Dallas, TX 75231

Finally, a brief point about nonpharmacological treatments. Some
interesting reports have shown that treatment with a placebo—a pill
that does not really do anything biologically—has actually lowered
blood pressure in some patients. That brings us to an interesting area:
the effect of the mind on BP and whether future treatments might be
psychologically oriented to a large extent. Whether the reductions
caused by placebo treatments are temporary or permanent remains to be
seen, but the role of the mind in controlling the body is one of the most
exciting avenues open to us.

The control of blood pressure will certainly change throughout your
lifetime, so keeping up with current knowledge is useful. And
underscore the word *lifetime*, because that is exactly what blood
pressure control is about: a lifetime project for increasing your lifetime.
That is the subject of Chapter 10. First, some frequently asked
questions concerning advances in hypertensive therapy:

Q: What's the big deal about continued research? It sounds like the
hypertension problem is pretty well wrapped up.

A: As mentioned, we have come a long way but there is a long way
to go. A small number of patients have blood pressure that still cannot
be controlled, and we must uncover more powerful and specific agents
for them.

Q: Is that the biggest problem—the people who do not respond to
medication?

A: In terms of numbers, no. The biggest problems are (1) the people
who do not seek treatment in the first place and (2) patients who do not
comply with treatment. We hope that public education and awareness
will, in the future, take care of problem number one. To a certain

extent, simpler delivery systems will help deal with the second difficulty.

Q: You mentioned that patients who dropped out of therapy several years ago would be more satisfied with modern treatments. I stopped my treatment but I am afraid to go back to my doctor because he will think I am a jerk.

A: A common problem. Lots of people—including some doctors, by the way—have slacked off on their treatment program. Your doctor will not think you are a jerk, but he or she will express disapproval of what you have done. The doctor *has* to take that attitude; he or she cannot pat every patient on the back and say, "That's okay, it happens to all of us," because—for some patients—this will minimize the perceived danger of hypertension, and that patient could drop out of treatment again.

[10]
Lifelong
Blood Pressure
Control

Treating the "silent killer" is a lifelong affair for both the patient and the doctor. Hypertension is not like 90 percent of illnesses treated in a doctor's office—acute, self-limiting illnesses. A strep throat will be cured with a prescription of an antibiotic; that is all there is to it. The problem is solved, and everybody is happy.

Hypertension, though, is long term, and it changes in nature and severity. Many patients feel that once they see a doctor and get on a blood pressure medication, the treatment will stay the same forever. That is simply not the case.

- The type of drug needed may change.
- The hypertension may become more severe or (less commonly) less severe all by itself.
- You may elect to try weight loss, exercise, and stress control in an effort to lower your dosage or eliminate drug treatment entirely.
- A new drug may treat your problem more effectively and with fewer side effects.
- The cause of your hypertension may change.

Hypertension is a problem that needs to be treated day by day, year to year. It is similar to alcoholism in the respect that once you are a hypertensive, you are always a hypertensive. Even if the blood pressure is under control, the potential for losing control is there. Just because BP goes down for a period of hours, days, or months, in most cases of essential hypertension a particular sequence of events could trigger it again.

If you understand this and accept this, you have a good start toward lifelong control. You have learned to think of hypertension not as a disease that will not be cured, but rather as a disease in which the effects and symptoms can be reduced. This is a helpful approach in understanding that blood pressure can skyrocket—given the right circumstances—even if you are taking medication.

There are, of course, certain situations where high blood pressure can be cured, such as removal of a tumor or repair of a renal artery. However, these cases do not relate to essential hypertension, the most common form of the disease.

Like it or not, high blood pressure is a part of your life, and you have to learn to live with it. To express it in the most blunt terms, it is a lot easier to learn to live with hypertension than with a stroke or with heart failure.

Getting Control of Your Life

The cause of hypertension is something like a bubbling cauldron—filled with bits and pieces of diet, daily life, and other medical problems—so it is important that you conquer the variables that can be under control. You cannot change the genetic makeup that predisposed you to the illness, but you can clamp down on other contributing factors. This has to be done over a *lifetime*.

As a case in point, it is not good enough for you to abstain from salty foods at a Christmas party but have two cups of salty soup every day for lunch. Treatment of hypertension extends to more than special situations or times when you feel ill. Hypertension is with you twenty-four hours a day for the rest of your life.

Conversely, if you pay close attention to your diet through the year but break down and eat some salty cheese at the Christmas party, you are not in imminent danger of keeling over at the hors d'oeuvre table with a stroke. Everything must be evaluated in light of *long-term* effects.

It is hard work, but for motivation you should pay close attention to your aunts and uncles who have had strokes at early ages and resolve that it will not happen to you. Learn from the mistakes of others and from your own mistakes. Evaluate what lack of compliance means to your life.

Also, make it a project to ascertain what happens to your blood pressure after eating a ham sandwich or having an argument with your spouse. Learn about your body because your body is *your* responsibility.

It is absolutely ludicrous to think that a doctor can take care of this problem with a short office visit and a few words of wisdom. *You* have to take control. Here is how:

Working with Your Doctor

Basically, you and your doctor must enter into an informal contract for blood pressure control. Each party has certain rights and responsibilities. The doctor has the right to know what is happening at all times, and you have the responsibility of telling the doctor about what is happening: whether you are having side effects, whether you are under great additional stress because you are having an extramarital affair, or whether you cannot afford to buy your drugs because you lost your money at the racetrack. What you tell your doctor will stay with your doctor. Ethically, physicians are sworn to uphold such confidentiality.

The doctor has the responsibility to inform the patient about drug treatment and its effects, and is obligated to give only whatever treatment is necessary. The doctor must, in all cases, carefully observe the benefit-risk ratio and observe the basic tenet of the Hippocratic Oath: First, do no harm.

Your family has a responsibility to you, too. They should not tempt you with salted food, and must not complain about how your diet affects them. A spouse should not smoke in front of a hypertensive who has given up the habit. Family members should be thoughtful and understanding of side effects you may have, and spouses should openly discuss problems involving sexual dysfunction.

Children have an obligation to take it a little easy on the old man if his blood pressure is up. They must try to avoid creating unduly stressful situations.

Finally, family members have an obligation to encourage weight loss, compliance with medications, and other aspects of a hypertensive's treatment program.

Ensuring Continuity of Care

A major problem encountered by hypertensives involves a lack of continuity in their care because they change doctors. Because our society is increasingly mobile, many patients move to different locations and never bother to have their medical records retrieved from their previous doctor. In that type of situation, patient and doctor have to start all over again with little information about prior treatment, illnesses, and so forth. Among other unpleasant possibilities, you run the risk of having the new doctor prescribe a medication that made you ill with side effects the first time it was tried.

Some patients shop from doctor to doctor within their home town. This is not a good idea; a patient needs one doctor to evaluate all medication and treatments, including those for hypertension. And you need a central place where all your records can be located in a hurry.

To once again repeat a common theme, with the many specialists you may see, there must be *one* coordinator of all your treatment and medication. Do not assume that the neurologist treating you for a stroke will be taking care of your blood pressure.

The continuity-of-care theme leads to the issue of the increasing complication of chemical agents in our everyday life. While a family physician can monitor your entire drug intake to check for adverse interactions, you also have to be aware of the nonprescription chemicals you put into your body. Over-the-counter decongestants, cough medicines, and diet pills may contain ingredients that can aggravate hypertension. Federal law requires that such drugs be labeled if they are contraindicated for use in patients with high blood pressure. The label will state that physician approval should be sought before taking the medication. Just to double-check, also keep an eye out for any drug that has the syllable "fed," such as Actifed, Novafed, or Sudafed.

Avoid the use of stimulants and be absolutely certain to steer clear of stimulants such as cocaine or, for that matter, any illicit drugs.

Monitoring Blood Pressure

We mentioned earlier that you should get a feel for how foods and activities affect your blood pressure. This is best accomplished by self-monitoring.

Learning to take your own blood pressure is an excellent option for some, but not all, blood pressure patients. Some people simply get so worked up over the idea of taking their blood pressure that the blood pressure goes up reflexively. In extreme cases, nervous people can develop a virtual hypertensive neurosis—a fear of and obsession with their blood pressure.

But for most people, self-monitoring is a fine idea. In fact, some studies have shown that self-monitoring tends to reduce BP. There are four major benefits:

- You can see how your blood pressure responds to factors in your life.
- You can gain encouragement by seeing your blood pressure fall.
- You can get to the doctor if something goes wrong.
- Your doctor will have an accurate and information-packed diary from which he or she can adjust your treatment and medication.

When to Take Your Blood Pressure

To start, you will probably want to check on your blood pressure three times a day or more. Experiment. Take the cuff with you to work; measure your blood pressure right before a meeting. Measure your blood pressure after dinner, after breakfast, right after you awaken, during the middle of the night if you wake up and have nothing else to do. *Write down* the results and the time, make a note of what you were doing at the time of the reading, and indicate how you felt—physically and mentally—at the time. A sample page for a blood pressure log is provided in Appendix D, and you and your doctor may find such a format useful for keeping track of your readings.

See if increases in your blood pressure seem associated with any symptoms you might have. Do this for two weeks or so, and show the readings to your doctor. The physician might decide that the introduction of an additional medication or a change in medication is in order.

Continue the monitoring, but as you get more used to the process, stop taking measurements at times when the blood pressure reading is relatively stable. But do take your blood pressure at times when it typically shoots up. And take a reading five or six hours after taking your medication.

The goal is to identify the factors that make your blood pressure rise so you can work to control them. Are those two cups of coffee in the morning responsible for your rise in blood pressure from 7 A.M. to 10 A.M.? Then they might have to be eliminated. Does your blood pressure remain high? Tell your doctor, because a different prescription might be more effective. Has your blood pressure steadily dropped because you have lost weight and stayed on your low-salt diet? Tell your doctor, because you now may be able to cut back on your medication.

Eventually, most patients settle into a routine of measuring their blood pressure about three times a week, or more often if there is an unusual event, such as an illness or drug side effects.

If you cannot take your own blood pressure or do not want to, there are other options. Often, your workplace or school will have a nurse who can take your pressure. Community service centers and health fairs frequently offer this service.

How to Take Your Blood Pressure

Any standard sphygmomanometer can be used. We have pictured one made by Tycos, but similar meters are available from many manufacturers, including Trimline, Propper, and Baumanometer. Just make sure you take the device to your doctor and have him or her:

- Watch you take your blood pressure to be sure your method is right.
- Take your blood pressure with the office sphygmomanometer to check on the accuracy of your instrument.

The newer digital blood pressure cuffs are very good alternatives. They are available from many manufacturers, including Pollenex, Timex, Bristoline, Nelkin, and Norelco (pictured in Figure 9). Some give a visual and an auditory reading: The machine beeps to tell you blood pressure is rising. Most digital machines also include a pulse-rate read-out. Your pulse rate is useful for your doctor to know, and you should consider taking your pulse and writing it into your blood pressure diary. Your pulse rate could be affected, for example, by antihypertensive medications, and your doctor will want to know this.

To take your pulse, simply place the first three fingers of your right hand on your left wrist, near the base of the thumb. Press down gently

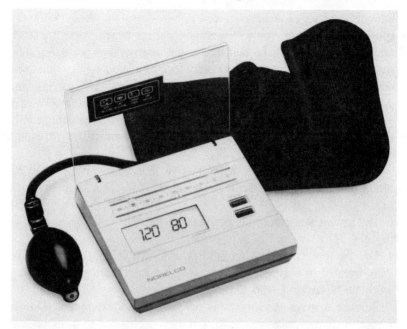

Figure 9. A Digital Blood Pressure Meter. This model also includes a pulse-rate read-out. (Photo courtesy of North American Philips Corp.)

until you feel the pulsing of your radial artery; count the beats for a minute or count them for thirty seconds and multiply by two.

Now, getting back to the instruments themselves, either a digital or standard sphygmomanometer is all right, just as long as your doctor checks it out. There is no compelling reason for an individual to buy a very expensive cuff, because the expensive models, designed for health care professionals, are not necessarily more accurate—they are just more durable. Much of the expense stems from the fact that they are designed to be used perhaps twenty times a day. In the same way, the price of digital machines will vary depending on whether you buy a standard model or one with fancy options, such as a print-out of your reading, and higher price does not necessarily reflect greater accuracy.

Blood pressure kits come with directions. The directions for the digital models will vary according to the hardware, but using a cuff and stethoscope is pretty much a standardized operation. Each unit will have its own set of directions, and be sure to follow them. With any sphygmomanometer, you will simply be placing the cuff over the upper arm, inflating it until the dial reads well over your expected systolic reading, then listening with the stethoscope over the artery as you undo the valve and deflate the cuff. The most important part of the procedure, and one that we illustrate here, is finding the artery. It is located where the finger points in Figure 10. Indeed, you can actually feel the artery if you probe deeply. Be sure the arrow on the cuff points to the artery.

When deflating the cuff, listen for the first time you can hear the blood pulsing and note the reading on the dial. That is the systolic reading.

The instant you can no longer hear the pulsing, note the reading on the dial. That is the diastolic reading.

The process takes practice and is awkward at first. The position demonstrated in Figure 11 shows a good posture from which you can work the valve and read the dial.

Be sure to save the directions on your individual model. Do not forget to demonstrate your cuff and your technique to your doctor.

Now It Is Up to You

This brings us to the conclusion of the book, and the most important point of our exploration of high blood pressure and how to beat it.

YOU MUST TAKE THE RESPONSIBILITY
FOR MANAGING YOUR OWN BLOOD PRESSURE.

All too often in medicine, patients cannot alter their disease and its prognosis; there is not all that much that they as individuals can do to alter the ultimate result of their diseases. They are almost entirely in the hands of doctors and hospitals.

That is not the case with hypertension. Mother Nature has gotten confused and she is trying to upset the fine balance within you. Do not let her. Stand up and fight back. You can!

Lose weight, exercise, watch your salt, and learn to cope with stress. You will be on the road to good health and normal pressure. Let your doctor provide you with the pharmacological ammunition you need.

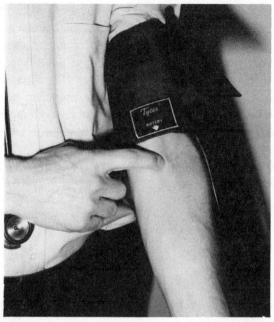

Figure 10. Locating the Artery. (Photo courtesy of Tycos Laboratories, Inc.)

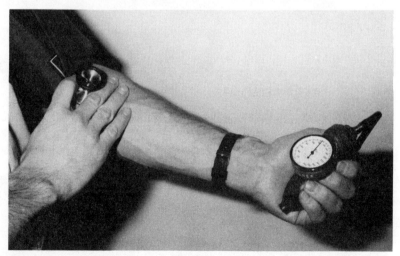

Figure 11. Taking the Reading. (Photo courtesy of Tycos Laboratories, Inc.)

And take your medicine. Do not stop if you "feel better." In the event the medicine creates side effects that bother you a great deal, tell your doctor and team up with him or her in the effort to find a suitable agent. Keep all your appointments and follow your doctor's advice.

It is true that you cannot cure yourself of this disease. Hypertension—even if you get your reading down to normal or near-normal—will always be lurking around the corner. But the odds are overwhelming that you *can control it*. You, personally, have the power to affect the course of this illness.

Conquer it.

Don't let it conquer you.

Appendixes

Appendix A. Low Sodium Diet

GENERAL INSTRUCTIONS

Your diet plan primarily uses foods which are prepared without salt and stresses the use of foods that are low in natural sodium.

Eat regularly as shown in your basic meal plan.

Select a variety of foods and do not add salt.

Carefully read the labels of all prepared foods. Look not only for salt, but also for bicarbonate of soda (baking soda), baking powder, MSG, and sodium compounds such as sodium benzoate, sodium citrate, etc. Most frozen dinners, instant dinner mixes, sauces, canned foods (except fruits and fruit juices) and prepared foods contain salt unless they are especially prepared for sodium-restricted diets and labeled as such.

Eat only the amount of List II foods specified in your basic meal plan. These foods are moderately high in sodium.

Choose a good source of Vitamin C daily. They are citrus fruits, strawberries, broccoli, brussels sprouts, papaya, and cantaloupes.

Choose a good source of Vitamin A every other day. These are dark green or yellow fruits and vegetables.

Water varies in sodium content from one area to another. Check with your local water supplier and if the water in your area contains more than 20 mg. sodium per quart, bottled water should be used. The use of water-softeners may add significant amounts of sodium to the water supply.

Avoid medicines, laxatives, and salt substitutes unless prescribed by physician.

Basic Meal Plan	Sample Menu	Calories	Sodium mg.	Cholesterol mg.	Special Instructions
BREAKFAST	**BREAKFAST**				**FOR WEIGHT CONTROL**
1 serving fruit or juice—List I	½ grapefruit	40	1		1. Follow a regular exercise program as directed by your physician.
1 serving cereal—List I	1 cup Puffed rice cereal (enriched) with	60	tr.		
1 serving nonfat milk—List II	1 cup nonfat milk	80	124.6	5	2. Avoid the use of wine, beer, or other alcoholic beverages.
1 serving fruit—List I	1 small banana	120	1		
1 serving salt-free bread—List I	1 slice salt-free whole wheat toast	61	5		3. Use only unsweetened or fresh fruits for desserts; avoid sugar, concentrated sweets, regular jelly and jams, regular soft drinks, etc. Artificial sweetener may be used.
1 serving fat—List I	1 tsp. unsalted margarine	34	—		
1 serving sweets—List I	1 tsp. jam	18	0.8		
Beverage	Coffee or tea	2	2		

NOON MEAL	**NOON MEAL**			
2 oz. cooked fresh meat—List II	2 oz. unsalted roasted chicken (light meat)	95	36	68
2 servings salt-free bread—List I	2 slices salt-free white bread and	124	5	3
1 serving fat—List I	1 tsp. salt-free mayonnaise with	33	—	
	lettuce (3 small leaves)	2	1	
1 serving vegetable—List I				
1 serving fruit—List I	1 box (1½ oz.) raisins	124	12	
1 serving fruit—List I	½ medium apple	40	1	
1 serving nonfat milk—List II	1 cup nonfat milk	80	124.6	5
EVENING MEAL	**EVENING MEAL**			
1 serving vegetables—List I	1 cup chopped fresh spinach	14	39	
1 serving vegetables—List I	½ medium tomato	11	1.5	
2 servings fat—List I	2 Tbsp. oil and vinegar dressing	166	1	
1 serving salt-free bread—List I	1 slice salt-free whole wheat bread	61	5	
1 serving fat—List I	1 tsp. unsalted margarine	34	—	
1 serving wine—List I (optional)	7 oz. wine	173	10.2	
4 oz. cooked fresh meat—List II	4 oz. broiled lean steak	234	67.8	103
1 serving vegetable—List I	1 baked potato	188	6	
2 servings fat—List I	2 Tbsp. sour cream	57	12	16
1 serving vegetable—List I	6 asparagus spears	18	1	
1 serving vegetable—List I	½ cup cooked rhubarb with sugar	191	2.5	
1 serving dessert—List II	½ cup ice cream	129	42	26
	Beverage Coffee or Tea	2	2	
BEDTIME	**BEDTIME**			
1 serving fruit—List I	1 medium orange	64	1	
	Total:	**2255**	**505**	**226**

4. Limit breads and cereals to 4 servings per day.
5. Limit margarine and other fats to 4 servings per day.
6. Avoid the use of potatoes or other starchy vegetables (including corn, lima beans, sweet potatoes, dried peas and beans)

SODIUM VARIATIONS

1. To convert diet to 1000mg sodium replace the 4 servings of salt-free bread with regular bread.
2. To convert diet to 2000mg sodium replace salt-free bread with 4 serving regular bread, replace salt-free margarine with regular margarine, and replace salt-free cereal with regular cereal, 1 cup maximum.

191

Adapted by the authors from "Sodium Restricted Diet Plan"; diet reference appears courtesy of the copyright owner © Carnation Company, Los Angeles, California.

Appendix A, *continued*. Substitution Lists for Low Sodium Diet

LIST I: FOODS WITH LOW SODIUM CONTENT—These foods may be used as desired unless calories are also restricted.

All fruit and fruit juices

All fresh or frozen vegetables except those in LIST II or LIST III

BREAD & CEREALS:	Puffed wheat/rice or shredded wheat
	Most hot, unsalted cereals
	Salt-free breads
	Pearl barley, rice, noodles, macaroni, spaghetti
	Popcorn, unsalted

FATS:	Sweet butter	Salt-free mayonnaise
	Unsalted margarine	Sour cream
	Vegetable oils	Nuts, unsalted
MISC:	Vinegar	Honey & syrup
	Wines	Sugar
	Jams or jellies	

Herbs and spices which do not contain salt or MSG (monosodium glutamate)

Special salt-free foods (read the label to determine milligram level per serving—under 15 mg. per serving foods may be used as desired)

LIST II: FOODS WITH MODERATE SODIUM CONTENT—These foods must be limited in amounts as specified.

MILK:	Limit to 2 cups Daily.
EGGS:	Limit to 1 per day.
DESSERTS:	Limit to one choice per day—serving portion as indicated.
	Cake—1½ oz.
	Cookies, assorted—1 oz.
	Gelatin—½ cup
	Ice Cream—½ cup
	Regular cooked puddings such as tapioca, rice, etc.—½ cup
	Sherbet—½ cup

*Meat/fish/fowl (other than those in List III)—Limit to 6 oz. cooked weight daily.

VEGETABLES:	Limit to one choice per day—½ cup serving only (fresh, frozen or salt-free canned)

Beets	Frozen Lima Beans
Beet greens	Frozen peas
Carrots	Kale
Chard	Mustard greens
Dandelion greens	Turnips, white
Celery	

*Fresh crab, lobster, shrimp, scallops, brains, kidneys, and frozen fish which have been flumed in brine contain higher amounts of sodium than other fresh meats. These foods should be chosen infrequently.

LIST III: FOODS WITH HIGH SODIUM CONTENT—These foods should be avoided.

MILK:
Buttermilk

CHEESE:
All excepting special low sodium cheese or low sodium cottage cheese.

MEATS/FISH/ FOWL:
Bacon, ham, frankfurters, sausages, bologna, luncheon meats; canned, salted, dried, smoked or pickled meat, fish or poultry. Herring, caviar, regular canned tuna & salmon, anchovies, sardines and salted cod. Canned crab, shrimp, lobster and oysters. Salt pork, chipped or corned beef, brain, kidney, meats koshered by salting. Regular peanut butter.

VEGETABLES:
Sauerkraut, olives, pickles, regular canned vegetables and canned vegetable juices. Any vegetable prepared in brine.

FATS:
Salted butter or margarine, commercial salad dressings and regular mayonnaise, bacon fat, salted nuts, canned gravies.

BREADS & CEREALS:
Regular and yeast breads and rolls prepared with salt, dry cereals other than those listed in List I, regular pancakes, muffins, biscuits, cornbread, crackers and mixes. Potato chips, corn chips, pretzels, salted popcorn, etc. Quick cooking cereals if a sodium compound has been added in processing. Cornmeal and self-rising flour.

SOUPS:
All regular canned soups, soup mixes, broth, bouillon, consomme, commercial bouillon cubes, powders or liquids.

DESSERTS:
Instant puddings, pie crust unless prepared without salt, desserts in excess of the amount allowed in List II.

BEVERAGES:
Dutch process cocoa, soft drinks or beer which have been bottled in areas with high sodium content in their water supplies.

CONDIMENTS:
Salt, seasonings which contain salt or monosodium glutamate, worcestershire sauce, soy sauce, meat tenderizers, regular catsup, chili sauce, barbecue sauce, horseradish sauce, etc. Pickles, relishes and olives.

Appendix B. Reducing Diet

GENERAL INSTRUCTIONS

Effective and sustained weight reduction can best be achieved through a regular plan of diet and exercise. The principles of the Reducing Diet Plan are as follows:

Eat regularly—do not omit a meal.

Follow a regular exercise program as directed by your physician. Between meal snacks should be chosen from the free list.

Vary the sample menu by choosing different foods as offered in the indicated substitution lists on the back of the diet. Eat those foods in the measured amounts indicated. Noon and evening basic meal plans may be interchanged when desired.

Choose a good source of Vitamin C daily. They are citrus fruits, strawberries, broccoli, brussels sprouts, papaya, and cantaloupe.

Choose a good source of Vitamin A every other day. These are dark green or yellow fruits and vegetables.

Broiling, roasting, steaming, boiling, or baking methods of food preparation are preferable. Avoid the use of fats and oils except in the amounts allowed. Avoid sugar, honey, concentrated sweets, pies, cakes, pastry, rich desserts, regular soft drinks and alcoholic beverages.

Basic Meal Plan 1200 Calories	Sample Menu	Calories	Special Instructions
See substitution lists for other allowable foods.			
BREAKFAST	**BREAKFAST**		☐ 1000 Calories: Omit 1 serving nonfat milk, 1 serving starch and 1 serving fat per day from basic meal plan.
1 serving fruit—List 3	1 grapefruit half	40	
1 serving starch—List 4	1 oz. enriched concentrate cereal	107	
1 serving nonfat milk—List 7	1 cup nonfat milk	80	
Miscellaneous—List 1	Sugar substitute	—	
Miscellaneous—List 1	Black Coffee	2	

194

NOON MEAL

2 measures meat/fish/fowl/cheese—List 5	
1 serving starch—List 4	
2 servings fruit—List 3	
½ serving nonfat milk—List 7	

NOON MEAL

2 oz. Cheddar cheese	223
5 small whole wheat crackers	57
1 medium apple	86
½ cup nonfat milk	40

EVENING MEAL

1 serving vegetable—List 1	
Miscellaneous—List 1	
4 measures meat/fish/fowl/cheese—List 5	
Miscellaneous—List 1	
1 serving starch—List 4	
1 serving fat—List 6	
1 serving vegetable—List 1	
Dessert—List 1	
Miscellaneous—List 1	

EVENING MEAL

1 cup fresh spinach salad	14
1 Tbsp. low calorie French dressing	15
4 oz. Broiled Halibut garnished with	205
1 lemon wedge	4
½ cup steamed rice with	112
1 tsp. margarine	34
6 asparagus spears	18
½ cup dietetic gelatin	8
Hot Tea	2

BEDTIME

2 servings fruit—List 3	
6 oz. nonfat milk—List 7	

BEDTIME

1 small banana		110
6 oz. nonfat milk		60
	total	1217

Adapted by the authors from "Reducing Diet Plan"; diet reference appears courtesy of the copyright owner © Carnation Company, Los Angeles, California.

195

Appendix B, *continued*. Substitution Lists for Reducing Diet

LIST 1 FREE FOOD LIST—These foods may be used as often as desired provided cream, sugar or honey, or fat is NOT added to them.

Miscellaneous
Coffee or Tea
Clear broth
Bouillon
Beverages, artificially sweetened containing less than 5 calories per 8 ounces
Jelly, artificially sweetened
Sugar substitute

Parsley
Herbs
Spices
Seasonings
Flavorings
Vinegar
Mustard
Horseradish
Salad dressing (dietetic)

Desserts & fruits
Cranberries
Lemons
Gelatin, unsweetened
Rennet tablets

Juices
Lemon juice
Tomato Juice
Vegetable juice

Vegetables
Asparagus
Bean sprouts
Beet greens
Broccoli
Brussels sprouts
Cabbage (all kinds)
Cauliflower
Celery
Chard
Chicory

Collard greens
Cucumbers
Dandelion greens
Escarole
Eggplant
Green beans
Kale
Lettuce (all kinds)
Mushrooms
Mustard greens

Okra
Peppers (green or red)
Radishes
Sauerkraut
Spinach
Squash, summer
Tomatoes
Turnip greens
Watercress
Wax beans

LIST 2 OTHER VEGETABLES—Limit these vegetables to one ½ cup serving per day (approximately 36 calories per serving)

Artichokes
Beets

Carrots
Onions

Peas, green
Pumpkin

Rutabaga
Squash, winter

Turnips

LIST 3 FRUITS AND FRUIT JUICES—May be fresh, cooked, dried, frozen or canned—NO SUGAR OR SYRUP (approximately 40 calories per serving or amounts indicated)

Fruits
Apple, medium—½
Applesauce—½ cup
Apricots, medium, fresh—2
Apricots, dried halves—4
Banana, small—½
Blackberries—1 cup
Blueberries—⅔ cup
Boysenberries—1 cup
Cantaloupe, medium—¼

Cherries, large—10
Dates—2
Figs, fresh, large—1
Figs, dried—1
Fruit cocktail, canned—½ cup
Grapefruit, small—½
Grapes—12
Honeydew melon—⅛

Mango, small—½
Nectarine, small—1
Orange, small—1
Papaya, medium—⅓
Peach, medium, fresh—1
Peach, canned—½ cup
Pear, dried halves—2
Pear, small fresh—1
Pear, canned—½ cup

Pear, dried halves—2
Pineapple—½ cup
Plums, medium, fresh—2
Prunes, dried—2
Raisins, dried, Tbsp.—2
Raspberries—1 cup
Strawberries—1 cup
Tangerine, large—1
Watermelon, cubed—1 cup

Juices
Apple—⅓ cup
Grape—¼ cup
Grapefruit—½ cup
Orange—½ cup
Pineapple—⅓ cup
Prune—¼ cup

LIST 4 STARCHES (approximately 70 calories per serving of amounts indicated)

Breads:
White, whole wheat or rye—1 slice
Bagel—½
Biscuit or muffin—1 (2" diameter)
Bun, hamb. or hot dot (8 to the pound)—½
Cornbread (1½" cube)—1
English muffin—½

Crackers
Graham (2½" sq.)—2
Melba toast—4
Oyster (½ cup)—20
Saltine—5
Round, thin—6
Ry-Krisp—3
Tortilla (6" dia.)—1
Wheat crackers—5

Cereals
Hot cereal—½ cup
Dry flakes—⅔ cup
Dry puffed—1½ cups
Rice or grits, cooked—½ cup
Spaghetti, macaroni, noodles or other pastas, cooked—½ cup

Vegetables
Beans or peas, dry cooked (lima, navy, kidney, blackeyed split, etc.)—½ cup
Beans, baked (no pork)—¼ cup
Corn—⅓ cup or ½ med ear
Potatoes, white (1 small)—½ cup
Potatoes, sweet or yams—¼ cup
Popcorn, popped (no butter)—1 cup

LIST 5 MEATS, FISH, FOWL—The following meats and meat substitutes are lowest in calories (approximately 50 calories per amount indicated). Select them as often as possible. Choose lean, unmarbled cuts; trim off all visible fat; do not add fat in cooking.

Beef, dried chipped—1 oz.
Beef, lamb, pork, ham, veal LEAN ONLY, cooked—1 oz.
Liver—1 oz.

Poultry without skin, cooked—1 oz.
Fish, any except those listed below—1 oz.
Crab—¼ cup
Clams, shrimp, or oysters—5 medium

Scallops (12/lb.)—1 large
Tuna, packed in water—¼ cup
Salmon, pink canned—¼ cup
Cottage cheese—¼ cup

The following meats and meat substitutes are higher in calories (approximately 73 calories per amount indicated). Select them sparingly.

Medium-fat meat (beef, lamb, pork, veal), cooked—1 oz.
Cold Cuts—1 oz.
Frankfurters (8–9/lb.)—1
Vienna sausages—2
Cheese (brick, cheddar, roquefort, swiss, processed, etc.)—1 oz.

Duck—1 oz.
Goose—1 oz.
Poultry with skin—1 oz.

Egg, whole—1
Salmon, red canned or smoked—¼ cup
Sardines—3 medium
Tuna, packed in oil—¼ cup
Peanut butter—2 Tsp.

LIST 6 FATS (approximately 45 calories per amount indicated)

Avocado (4" diam.)—⅛
Bacon, crisp—1 slice
Butter, margarine—1 tsp.

Cream, sour—2 Tbsp.
Cream cheese—1 Tbsp.
Nuts—6 small

Dressing, french—1 Tbsp.
Mayonnaise—1 tsp.
Roquefort dressing—2 tsp.

1000 Island dressing—2 tsp.
Oil—1 tsp.
Olives—5 small

LIST 7 MILK EXCHANGES—Approximately 12 grams carbohydrate, 8 grams protein, trace fat, 80 calories per serving.

Nonfat Dry Milk (Liquid)—1 cup; (Dry)—⅓ cup
Buttermilk, fat free—1 cup
Yogurt, plain, made with nonfat milk—1 cup

Other—omit 1 fat exchange:
Lowfat milk—1 cup
Yogurt made with lowfat milk—1 cup

Other—omit 2 fat exchanges:
Whole milk—1 cup
Evaporated Milk—½ cup
Buttermilk made from whole milk—1 cup

Appendix C. Cholesterol Control Diet

GENERAL INSTRUCTIONS

Eat regularly as indicated on your sample menu. Servings of margarine and oils, breads and cereals, fruits or vegetables may be added or subtracted from the diet plan to adjust the calorie intake.

Choose fish, poultry, and other protein foods in List II (on back) often. Eat less beef, lamb, pork, regular cheese, and other foods in List IV which are extremely high in cholesterol. Limit meat, fish, or poultry servings to 6 oz. per day, as indicated in

your Basic Meal Plan.

Prepare foods with corn, cottonseed, soybean, or safflower oil and choose margarines which are polyunsaturated.

Choose a good source of Vitamin C daily. They are citrus fruits, strawberries, broccoli, brussels sprouts, papaya, and cantaloupe. Choose a good source of Vitamin A every other day. These are dark green or yellow fruits and vegetables.

Basic Meal Plan	**Sample Menu**	Calories	Chol. Mg.
See substitution lists for other allowable foods.			
BREAKFAST	**BREAKFAST**		
1 serving fruit or juice	1 grapefruit half	40	
1 serving cereal with	1 cup enriched dry cereal	60	
½ cup nonfat milk	½ cup nonfat milk	40	
2 servings bread	2 slices white toast	124	
2 servings margarine	2 tsp. margarine	68	
1 serving sweets	1 Tbsp. jam	54	
Beverage	Coffee without cream	2	2.5

198

NOON MEAL	**NOON MEAL**		
1 serving cooked vegetable	1 cup vegetable soup	78	
1 serving bread or crackers	4 saltine crackers	47	
1 serving fish or poultry	3 oz. roast turkey, white meat	150	
2 servings bread	2 slices white bread	124	65.5
2 servings margarine	2 tsp. margarine	68	
1 serving raw vegetable	3 carrot & 3 celery sticks	19	
1 serving fruit	1 medium apple	87	
1 serving nonfat milk	1 cup nonfat milk	80	5
Beverage	Tea or coffee without cream	2	
EVENING MEAL	**EVENING MEAL**		
1 serving meat, fish, fowl	3 oz. broiled halibut	154	
1 serving starchy vegetable	1 baked potato	188	54
1 serving bread	1 slice French bread	43	
3 servings margarine	3 tsp. margarine	102	
1 serving cooked vegetable	½ cup green beans	17	
2 servings raw vegetables	Large lettuce & tomato salad	23	
2 servings salad dressing	2 Tbsp. Italian dressing	166	
1 serving dessert	½ cup orange sherbet	129	
1 serving nonfat milk	1 cup nonfat milk	80	5
Beverage	Tea or coffee without cream	2	
BEDTIME	**BEDTIME**		
1 serving fruit	1 1½ oz. package of raisins	120	
1 serving nonfat milk	8 oz. nonfat milk	80	5
1 serving bread or crackers	2 graham crackers	65	

Total: 2212   137 mg.

Adapted by the authors from "Cholesterol Control Diet Plan for Normal Weight Patients"; diet reference appears courtesy of the copyright owner © Carnation Company, Los Angeles, California.

Appendix C, *continued*. Substitution Lists for Cholesterol Control Diet

LIST I — Foods of plant origin contain no cholesterol. These are fruits, vegetables, cereals, grains, nuts, and vegetable oils. However, choosing liquid or unsaturated vegetable oils, rather than "hydrogenated" (solid) vegetable oil products is sometimes recommended as these oils may have a cholesterol-lowering effect. Exceptions to this rule are coconut and olive oil.

LIST II — These animal-origin foods are low in cholesterol:

	Chol. mg.		Chol. mg.		Chol. mg.
3 oz cottage cheese	8	3 oz haddock	51	1 cup nonfat milk	5
3 oz chicken, white	67	3 oz halibut	51	1 cup buttermilk	5
3 oz cod	48	3 oz salmon	40	1 cup yogurt (low fat)	17
3 oz (bass, whiting, carp,		3 oz trout	47	Egg white	0
sole, pollack,		3 oz tuna	55		
pike, perch)	50-70	3 oz turkey, white	65		
3 oz flounder	43				

LIST III — These animal-origin foods are higher in cholesterol, but may still have a cholesterol-lowering effect because of their unsaturated or low-total fat content.

	Chol. mg.		Chol. mg.
3 oz chicken, dark	77	3 oz herring	82
3 oz crab	85	3 oz lobster	72
		3 oz turkey, dark	86

LIST IV — These animal-origin foods are high in cholesterol or may have a cholesterol-raising effect. They should be limited.

Food	Chol. mg.	Food	Chol. mg.	Food	Chol. mg.
3 oz beef	80	3 oz lamb	83	3 oz cheese, cheddar	84
3 oz brains	1,700	3 oz liver	372	3 oz cheese, Swiss	85
3 oz chicken gizzards	166	3 oz pork	76	3 oz cheese, American	77
3 oz heart	233	3 oz sardines	119	*3 oz clams	43
3 oz kidneys	683	3 oz sausage	53	*3 oz oysters	43
3 oz sweetbread	396	3 oz shrimp	128	*3 oz scallops	45
		3 oz veal	86		
1 cup milk, whole	34	1 Tbl. butter	35	1 Tbl. ½ & ½	6
1 egg (50 g), whole	252	1 Tbl. chicken fat	9	1 Tbl. sour cream	8
1 egg yolk (17 g)	252	1 Tbl. cream cheese	16	1 Tbl. whipping cream, unwhipped	20
		1 Tbl. lard	13		

LIST V — Cholesterol content of products which contain animal-origin foods.

Food	Chol. mg.	Food	Chol. mg.	Food	Chol. mg.
1 piece angel cake	0	1 muffin (40 g)	21	1 popover	59
1 piece yellow cake (75 g)	33	1 corn muffin (40 g)	28	1 waffle	119
1 piece sponge cake (66 g)	162	½ cup noodles	25	**1 Tbl. mayonnaise	10
1 cream puff (130 g)	188	⅛ apple pie	120		
½ cup custard	139	⅛ lemon pie	117		
½ cup ice cream (10% fat)	27	⅛ pumpkin pie	70		
½ cup ice milk	13	½ cup potato salad	81		
½ cup pudding (mix)	15	½ cup white sauce	17		

*Cholesterol accounts for only 30% of the total sterol in scallops and only 40% in oysters and clams. The other sterols in these shellfish require further study and may have nutritional significance.

**Imitation mayonnaise and mayonnaise made with safflower oil contain less cholesterol.

Appendix D. A Sample Page for a Blood Pressure Log

Date	Time (Enter time you take BP, pulse, and each dose of medicine)	Blood Pressure Reading	Pulse Rate	Name of Medicine Taken	How are you feeling now?	Special Comments, Remarks

Index